From the Mediterranean Sea to Your Plate

Fish for Compliments With These Delectable Fish & Seafood Recipes

By
Delia Bell

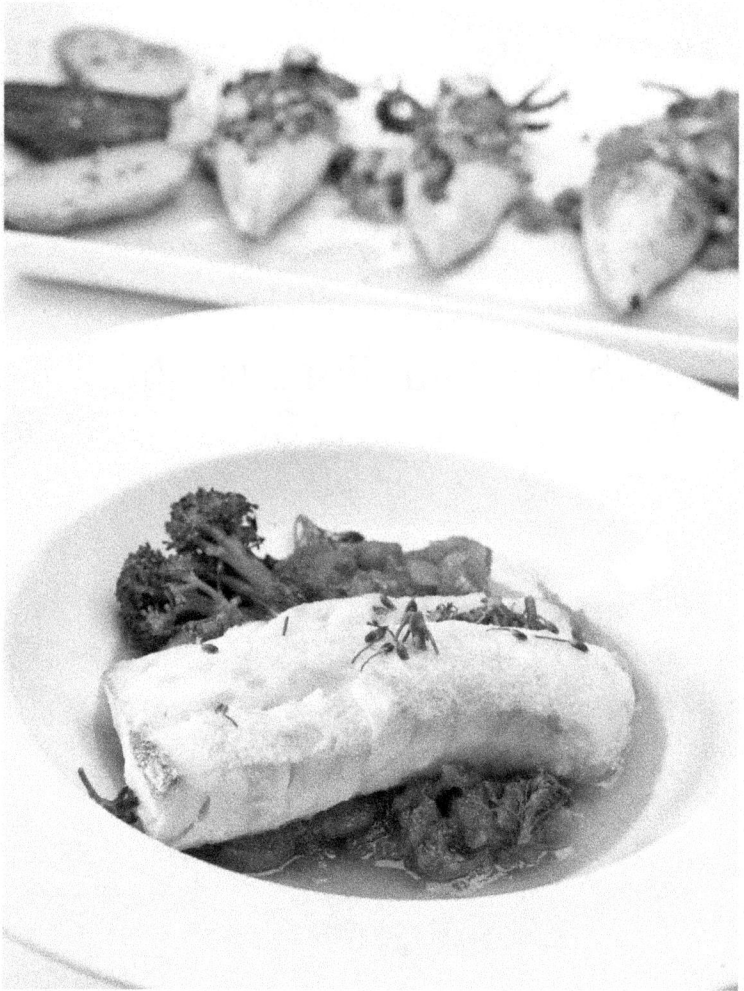

Table of Contents

INTRODUCTION

What is the Mediterranean Diet?

The Mediterranean diet is based on the diets of traditional eating habits from the 1960s of people from countries that surround the Mediterranean Sea, such as Greece, Italy, and Spain, and it encourages the consumption of fresh, seasonal, and local foods. The Mediterranean diet has become popular because individuals show low rates of heart disease, chronic disease, and obesity. The Mediterranean diet profile focuses on whole grains, good fats (fish, olive oil, nuts etc.), vegetables, fruits, fish, and very low consumption of any non-fish meat. Along with food, the Mediterranean diet emphasizes the need to spend time eating with family and physical activity. The Mediterranean diet is not a single prescribed diet, but rather a general food-based eating pattern, which is marked by local and cultural differences throughout the Mediterranean region.

The diet is generally characterized by a high intake of plant-based foods (e.g. fresh fruit and vegetables, nuts, and cereals) and olive oil, a moderate intake of fish and poultry, and low intakes of dairy products (mostly yoghurt and cheese), red and processed meats, and sweets. Wine is typically consumed in moderation and, normally, with a meal. A strong focus is placed on social and cultural aspects, such as communal mealtimes, resting after eating, and regular physical activity. Nowadays, however, the diet is no longer followed as widely as it was 30-50 years ago, as the diets of people living in these regions are becoming more 'Westernized' and higher in energy dense foods.

Benefits

The Mediterranean diet is not a weight loss, but increasing fiber intake and cutting out red meat, animal fats, and processed food may lead to weight loss. People who follow the diet may also have a lower risk of various diseases.

Heart health

In the 1950s, an American scientist, found that people living in the poorer areas of southern Italy had a lower risk of heart disease and death than those in wealthier parts of New York. Dr. Keys attributed this to diet. Since then, many studies have indicated that following a Mediterranean diet can help the body maintain healthy cholesterol levels and reduce the risk of high blood pressure and cardiovascular disease. The overall pattern of the Mediterranean diet is similar to their own dietary recommendations. A high proportion of calories on the diet come from fat, which can increase the risk of obesity. However, they also note that this fat is mainly unsaturated, which makes it a more healthful option than that from the typical American diet.

Protection from disease

The Mediterranean diet focuses on plant-based foods, and these are good sources of antioxidants.

The Mediterranean diet might offer protection from various cancers, and especially colorectal cancer. The reduction in risk may stem from the high intake of fruits, vegetables, and whole grains. By sticking to Mediterranean meals, people's levels of blood glucose and fats had decreased. During this time, there was also a lower incidence of stroke.

Diabetes

The Mediterranean diet may help prevent type 2 diabetes and improve markers of diabetes in people who already have the condition. Various other studies have concluded that following the Mediterranean diet can reduce the risk of type 2 diabetes and cardiovascular disease, which often occur together.

Food to eat

There is no single definition of the Mediterranean diet, but one group of scientists used the following as their 2015 basis of research.

Vegetables: Include 3 to 9 servings a day.

Fresh fruit: Up to 2 servings a day.

Cereals: Mostly whole grain from 1 to 13 servings a day.

Oil: Up to 8 servings of extra virgin (cold pressed) olive oil a day.

Fat — mostly unsaturated — made up 37% of the total calories. Unsaturated fat comes from plant sources, such as olives and avocado. The Mediterranean diet also provided 33 grams (g) of fiber a day. The baseline diet for this study provided around

2,200 calories a day. Typical ingredients. Here are some examples of ingredients that people often include in the Mediterranean diet.

Vegetables: Tomatoes, peppers, onions, eggplant, zucchini, cucumber, leafy green vegetables, plus others.
Fruits: Melon, apples, apricots, peaches, oranges, and lemons, and so on.
Legumes: Beans, lentils, and chickpeas.
Nuts and seeds: Almonds, walnuts, sunflower seeds, and cashews.
Unsaturated fat: Olive oil, sunflower oil, olives, and avocados.
Dairy products: Cheese and yogurt are the main dairy foods.
Cereals: These are mostly whole grain and include wheat and rice with bread accompanying many meals.
Fish: Sardines and other oily fish, as well as oysters and other shellfish. Poultry: Chicken or turkey.
Eggs: Chicken, quail, and duck eggs.
Drinks: A person can drink red wine in moderation.

The Mediterranean diet does not include strong liquor or carbonated and sweetened drinks. According to one definition, the diet limits red meat and sweets to less than 2 servings per week.

Food to avoid

Here's a list of foods you should generally limit while eating Mediterranean-style meals. Heavily processed foods. Let's be real: Many, many foods are processed to some degree. A can of beans has been processed, in the sense that the beans have been cooked before being canned. Olive oil has been processed, because olives have been turned into oil. But when we talk about limiting processed foods, this really means avoiding things like frozen meals with tons of sodium. You should also limit soda, desserts and candy. As the adage goes, if the ingredient list includes items that your great-grandparents wouldn't recognize as food, it's probably processed. If you're buying a packaged food that's as close to its whole-food form as possible — such as frozen fruit or veggies with nothing added — you're good to go.

Processed red meat

On the Mediterranean diet, you should minimize your intake of red meat, such as steak. What about processed red meat, such as hot dogs and bacon? You should avoid these foods or limit them as much as possible. A study published in BMJ found that regularly eating red meat, especially processed varieties, was associated with a higher risk of death. Butter. Here's another food that should be limited on the Mediterranean diet. Use olive oil instead, which has many heart health benefits and contains less saturated fat than butter. According to the USDA National Nutrient Database, butter has 7 grams of saturated fat per tablespoon, while olive oil has about 2 grams.

Refined grains

The Mediterranean diet is centered around whole grains, such as farro, millet, couscous and brown rice. With this eating style, you'll generally want to limit your intake of refined grains such as white pasta and white bread.

Alcohol

When you're following the Mediterranean diet, red wine should be your chosen alcoholic drink. This is because red wine offers health benefits, particularly for the heart. But it's important to limit intake of any type of alcohol to up to one drink per day for women, as well as men older than 65, and up to two drinks daily for men age 65 and younger. The amount that counts as a drink is 5 ounces of wine, 12 ounces of beer or 1.5 ounces of 80-proof liquor.

Tomato Cod Mix

Servings: 2

Cooking Time: 5.5 Hours

Ingredients:

- 1 teaspoon tomato paste
- 1 teaspoon garlic, diced
- 1 white onion, sliced
- 1 jalapeno pepper, chopped
- 1/3 cup chicken stock
- 7 oz Spanish cod fillet
- 1 teaspoon paprika
- 1 teaspoon salt

Directions:

1. Pour chicken stock in the saucepan.
2. Add tomato paste and mix up the liquid until homogenous.
3. Add garlic, onion, jalapeno pepper, paprika, and salt.
4. Bring the liquid to boil and then simmer it.
5. Chop the cod fillet and add it in the tomato liquid.
6. Close the lid and simmer the fish for 10 minutes over the low heat.
7. Serve the fish in the bowls with tomato sauce.

Nutrition Info:Per Serving:calories 113, fat 1.2, fiber 1.9, carbs 7.2, protein 18.9

Garlic Mussels

Servings: 4

Cooking Time: 10 Minutes

Ingredients:

- 1-pound mussels
- 1 chili pepper, chopped
- 1 cup chicken stock
- ½ cup milk
- 1 teaspoon olive oil
- 1 teaspoon minced garlic
- 1 teaspoon ground coriander
- ½ teaspoon salt
- 1 cup fresh parsley, chopped
- 4 tablespoons lemon juice

Directions:

1. Pour milk in the saucepan.

2. Add chili pepper, chicken stock, olive oil, minced garlic, ground coriander, salt, and lemon juice.

3. Bring the liquid to boil and add mussels.

4. Boil the mussel for 4 minutes or until they will open shells.

5. Then add chopped parsley and mix up the meal well.

6. Remove it from the heat.

Nutrition Info:Per Serving:calories 136, fat 4.7, fiber 0.6, carbs 7.5, protein 15.3

Mahi Mahi And Pomegranate Sauce

Servings: 4

Cooking Time: 10 Minutes

Ingredients:

- 1 and ½ cups chicken stock
- 1 tablespoon olive oil
- 4 mahi mahi fillets, boneless
- 4 tablespoons tahini paste
- Juice of 1 lime
- Seeds from 1 pomegranate
- 1 tablespoon parsley, chopped

Directions:

1. Heat up a pan with the oil over medium-high heat, add the fish and cook for 3 minutes on each side.
2. Add the rest of the ingredients, flip the fish again, cook for 4 minutes more, divide everything between plates and serve.

Nutrition Info: calories 224, fat 11.1, fiber 5.5, carbs 16.7, protein 11.4

Honey Balsamic Salmon

Servings: 2

Cooking Time: 3 Minutes

Ingredients:

- 2 salmon fillets
- 1/4 tsp red pepper flakes
- 2 tbsp honey
- 2 tbsp balsamic vinegar
- 1 cup of water
- Pepper
- Salt

Directions:

1. Pour water into the instant pot and place trivet in the pot.
2. In a small bowl, mix together honey, red pepper flakes, and vinegar.
3. Brush fish fillets with honey mixture and place on top of the trivet.
4. Seal pot with lid and cook on high for 3 minutes.
5. Once done, release pressure using quick release. Remove lid. 6. Serve and enjoy.

Nutrition Info: Calories 303 Fat 11 g Carbohydrates 17.6 g Sugar 17.3 g Protein 34.6 g Cholesterol 78 mg

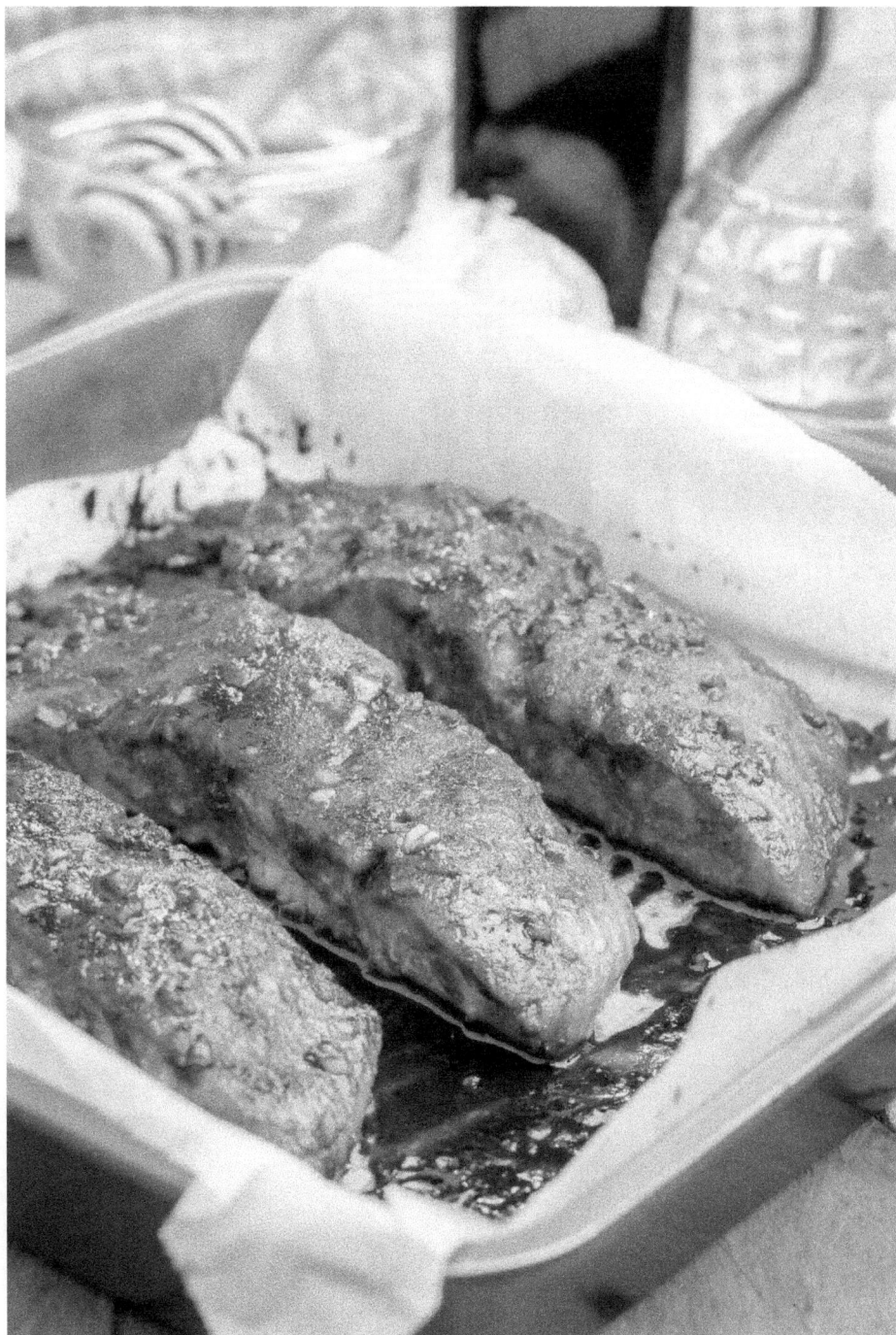

Sage Salmon Fillet

Servings: 1

Cooking Time: 25 Minutes

Ingredients:
- 4 oz salmon fillet
- ½ teaspoon salt
- 1 teaspoon sesame oil
- ½ teaspoon sage

Directions:

1. Rub the fillet with salt and sage.

2. Place the fish in the tray and sprinkle it with sesame oil.

3. Cook the fish for 25 minutes at 365F.

4. Flip the fish carefully onto another side after 12 minutes of cooking.

Nutrition Info:Per Serving:calories 191, fat 11.6, fiber 0.1, carbs 0.2, protein 22

Seafood Stew Cioppino

Servings: 6

Cooking Time: 40 Minutes

Ingredients:

- ¼ cup Italian parsley, chopped
- ¼ tsp dried basil
- ¼ tsp dried thyme
- ½ cup dry white wine like pinot grigio
- ½ lb. King crab legs, cut at each joint
- ½ onion, chopped
- ½ tsp red pepper flakes (adjust to desired spiciness)
- 1 28-oz can crushed tomatoes
- 1 lb. mahi mahi, cut into ½-inch cubes
- 1 lb. raw shrimp
- 1 tbsp olive oil
- 2 bay leaves
- 2 cups clam juice
- 50 live clams, washed
- 6 cloves garlic, minced
- Pepper and salt to taste

Directions:

1. On medium fire, place a stockpot and heat oil.
2. Add onion and for 4 minutes sauté until soft.

3. Add bay leaves, thyme, basil, red pepper flakes and garlic. Cook for a minute while stirring a bit.

4. Add clam juice and tomatoes. Once simmering, place fire to medium low and cook for 20 minutes uncovered.

5. Add white wine and clams. Cover and cook for 5 minutes or until clams have slightly opened.

6. Stir pot then add fish pieces, crab legs and shrimps. Do not stir soup to maintain the fish's shape. Cook while covered for 4 minutes or until clams
are fully opened; fish and shrimps are opaque and cooked.

7. Season with pepper and salt to taste.

8. Transfer Cioppino to serving bowls and garnish with parsley before serving.

Nutrition Info: Calories per Serving: 371; Carbs: 15.5 g; Protein: 62 g; Fat: 6.8 g

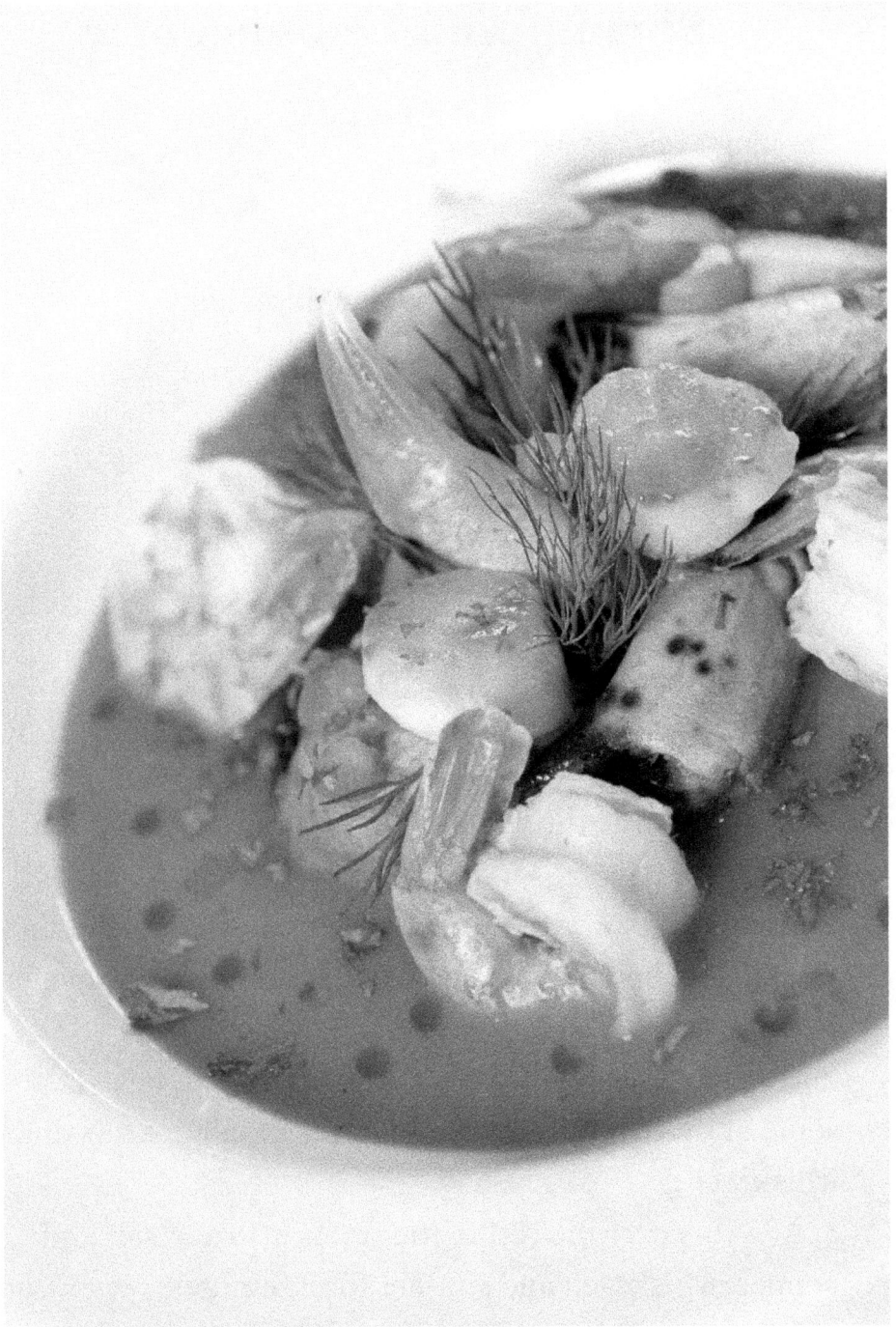

Shrimp And Lemon Sauce

Servings: 4

Cooking Time: 15 Minutes

Ingredients:

- 1 pound shrimp, peeled and deveined
- 1/3 cup lemon juice
- 4 egg yolks
- 2 tablespoons olive oil
- 1 cup chicken stock
- Salt and black pepper to the taste
- 1 cup black olives, pitted and halved
- 1 tablespoon thyme, chopped

Directions:

1. In a bowl, mix the lemon juice with the egg yolks and whisk well.

2. Heat up a pan with the oil over medium heat, add the shrimp and cook for 2 minutes on each side and transfer to a plate.

3. Heat up a pan with the stock over medium heat, add some of this over the egg yolks and lemon juice mix and whisk well.

4. Add this over the rest of the stock, also add salt and pepper, whisk well and simmer for 2 minutes.

5. Add the shrimp and the rest of the ingredients, toss and serve right away.

Nutrition Info: calories 237, fat 15.3, fiber 4.6, carbs 15.4, protein 7.6

Feta Tomato Sea Bass

Servings: 4

Cooking Time: 8 Minutes

Ingredients:
- 4 sea bass fillets
- 1 1/2 cups water
- 1 tbsp olive oil
- 1 tsp garlic, minced
- 1 tsp basil, chopped
- 1 tsp parsley, chopped
- 1/2 cup feta cheese, crumbled
- 1 cup can tomatoes, diced
- Pepper
- Salt

Directions:

1. Season fish fillets with pepper and salt.

2. Pour 2 cups of water into the instant pot then place steamer rack in the pot.

3. Place fish fillets on steamer rack in the pot.

4. Seal pot with lid and cook on high for 5 minutes.

5. Once done, release pressure using quick release. Remove lid.

6. Remove fish fillets from the pot and clean the pot.

7. Add oil into the inner pot of instant pot and set the pot on sauté mode.

8. Add garlic and sauté for 1 minute.

9. Add tomatoes, parsley, and basil and stir well and cook for 1 minute. 10. Add fish fillets and top with crumbled cheese and cook for a minute. 11. Serve and enjoy.

Nutrition Info: Calories 219 Fat 10.1 g Carbohydrates 4 g Sugar 2.8 g Protein 27.1 g Cholesterol 70 mg

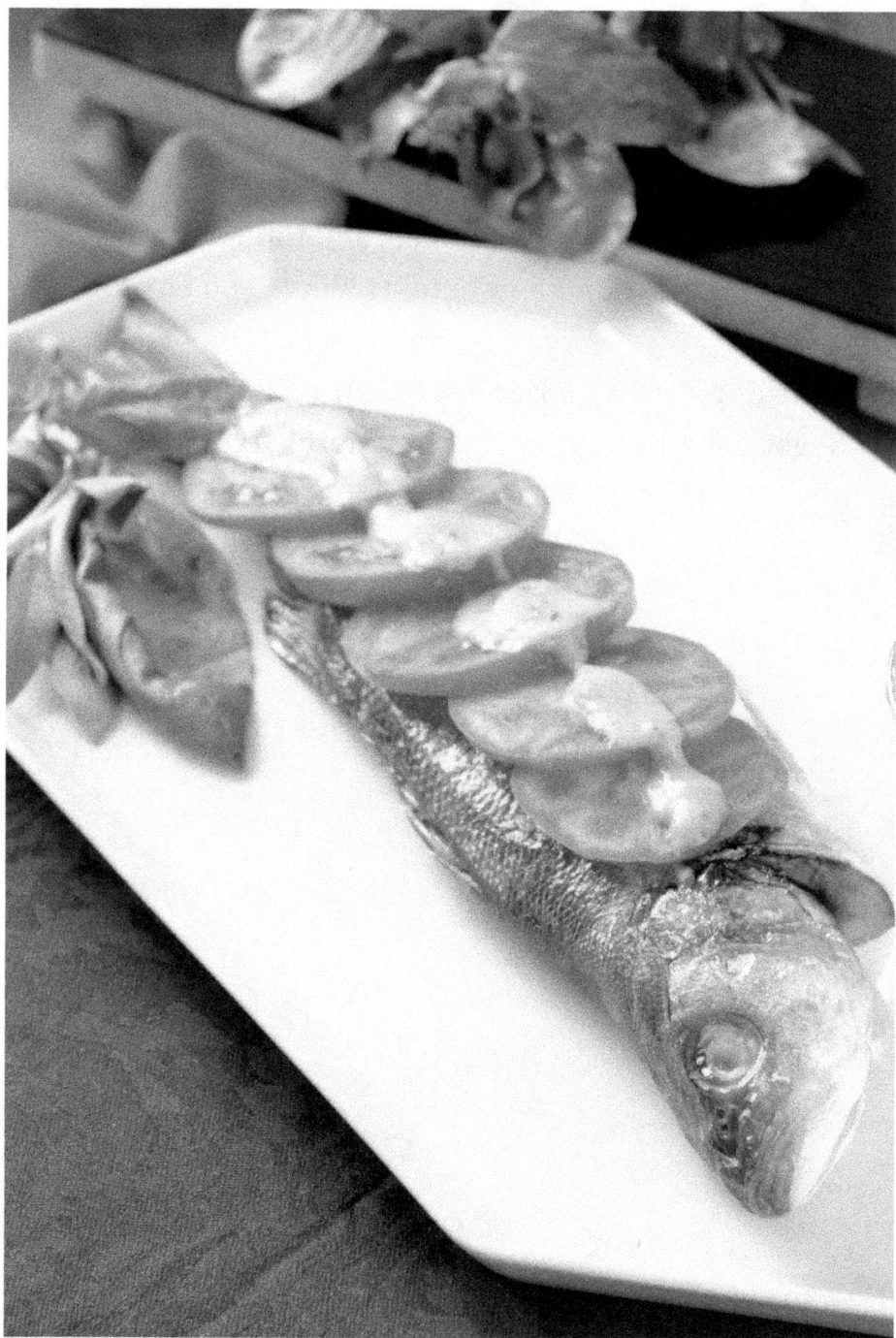

Salmon And Broccoli

Servings: 4

Cooking Time: 20 Minutes

Ingredients:

- 2 tablespoons balsamic vinegar
- 1 broccoli head, florets separated
- 4 pieces salmon fillets, skinless
- 1 big red onion, roughly chopped
- 1 tablespoon olive oil
- Sea salt and black pepper to the taste

Directions:

1. In a baking dish, combine the salmon with the broccoli and the rest of the ingredients, introduce in the oven and bake at 390 degrees F for 20 minutes.

2. Divide the mix between plates and serve.

Nutrition Info: calories 302, fat 15.5, fiber 8.5, carbs 18.9, protein 19.8

Halibut And Quinoa Mix

Servings: 4

Cooking Time: 12 Minutes

Ingredients:
- 4 halibut fillets, boneless
- 2 tablespoons olive oil
- 1 teaspoon rosemary, dried
- 2 teaspoons cumin, ground
- 1 tablespoons coriander, ground
- 2 teaspoons cinnamon powder
- 2 teaspoons oregano, dried
- A pinch of salt and black pepper
- 2 cups quinoa, cooked
- 1 cup cherry tomatoes, halved
- 1 avocado, peeled, pitted and sliced
- 1 cucumber, cubed
- ½ cup black olives, pitted and sliced
- Juice of 1 lemon

Directions:

1. In a bowl, combine the fish with the rosemary, cumin, coriander, cinnamon, oregano, salt and pepper and toss.

2. Heat up a pan with the oil over medium heat, add the fish, and sear for 2 minutes on each side.

3. Introduce the pan in the oven and bake the fish at 425 degrees F for 7 minutes.

4. Meanwhile, in a bowl, mix the quinoa with the remaining ingredients, toss and divide between plates.

5. Add the fish next to the quinoa mix and serve right away.

Nutrition Info: calories 364, fat 15.4, fiber 11.2, carbs 56.4, protein 24.5

Crab Stew

Servings: 2

Cooking Time: 13 Minutes

Ingredients:
- 1/2 lb lump crab meat
- 2 tbsp heavy cream
- 1 tbsp olive oil
- 2 cups fish stock
- 1/2 lb shrimp, shelled and chopped
- 1 celery stalk, chopped
- 1/2 tsp garlic, chopped
- 1/4 onion, chopped
- Pepper
- Salt

Directions:

1. Add oil into the inner pot of instant pot and set the pot on sauté mode.

2. Add onion and sauté for 3 minutes.

3. Add garlic and sauté for 30 seconds.

4. Add remaining ingredients except for heavy cream and stir well.

5. Seal pot with lid and cook on high for 10 minutes.

6. Once done, release pressure using quick release. Remove lid.

7. Stir in heavy cream and serve.

Nutrition Info: Calories 376 Fat 25.5 g Carbohydrates 5.8 g Sugar 0.7 g Protein 48.1 g Cholesterol 326 mg

Crazy Saganaki Shrimp

Servings: 4
Cooking Time: 10 Minutes

Ingredients:
- ¼ tsp salt
- ½ cup Chardonnay
- ½ cup crumbled Greek feta cheese
- 1 medium bulb. fennel, cored and finely chopped
- 1 small Chile pepper, seeded and minced
- 1 tbsp extra virgin olive oil
- 12 jumbo shrimps, peeled and deveined with tails left on
- 2 tbsp lemon juice, divided
- 5 scallions sliced thinly
- Pepper to taste

Directions:
1. In medium bowl, mix salt, lemon juice and shrimp.
2. On medium fire, place a saganaki pan (or large nonstick saucepan) and heat oil.
3. Sauté Chile pepper, scallions, and fennel for 4 minutes or until starting to brown and is already soft.
4. Add wine and sauté for another minute.
5. Place shrimps on top of fennel, cover and cook for 4 minutes or until shrimps are pink.

6. Remove just the shrimp and transfer to a plate.

7. Add pepper, feta and 1 tbsp lemon juice to pan and cook for a minute or until cheese begins to melt.

8. To serve, place cheese and fennel mixture on a serving plate and top with shrimps.

Nutrition Info: Calories per serving: 310; Protein: 49.7g; Fat: 6.8g; Carbs: 8.4g

Grilled Tuna

Servings: 3

Cooking Time: 6 Minutes

Ingredients:
- 3 tuna fillets
- 3 teaspoons teriyaki sauce
- ½ teaspoon minced garlic
- 1 teaspoon olive oil

Directions:

1. Whisk together teriyaki sauce, minced garlic, and olive oil.

2. Bruhs every tuna fillet with teriyaki mixture.

3. Preheat grill to 390F.

4. Grill the fish for 3 minutes from each side.

Nutrition Info:Per Serving:calories 382, fat 32.6, fiber 0, carbs 1.1, protein 21.4

Rosemary Salmon

Servings: 5

Cooking Time: 10 Minutes

Ingredients:
- 2-pound salmon fillet
- 2 tablespoons avocado oil
- 2 teaspoons fresh rosemary, chopped
- ½ teaspoon minced garlic
- ½ teaspoon dried cilantro
- ½ teaspoon salt
- 1 teaspoon butter
- ½ teaspoon white pepper

Directions:

1. Whisk together avocado oil, fresh rosemary, minced garlic, dried cilantro, salt, and white pepper.

2. Rub the salmon fillet with the rosemary mixture generously and leave fish in the fridge for 20 minutes to marinate.

3. After this, put butter in the saucepan or big skillet and melt it.

4. Then put heat on maximum and place a salmon fillet in the hot butter.

5. Roast it for 1 minute from each side.

6. After this, preheat grill to 385F and grill the fillet for 8 minutes (for 4 minutes from each side).

7. Cut the cooked salmon on the servings.

Nutrition Info:Per Serving:calories 257, fat 12.8, fiber 0.5, carbs 0.9, protein 35.3

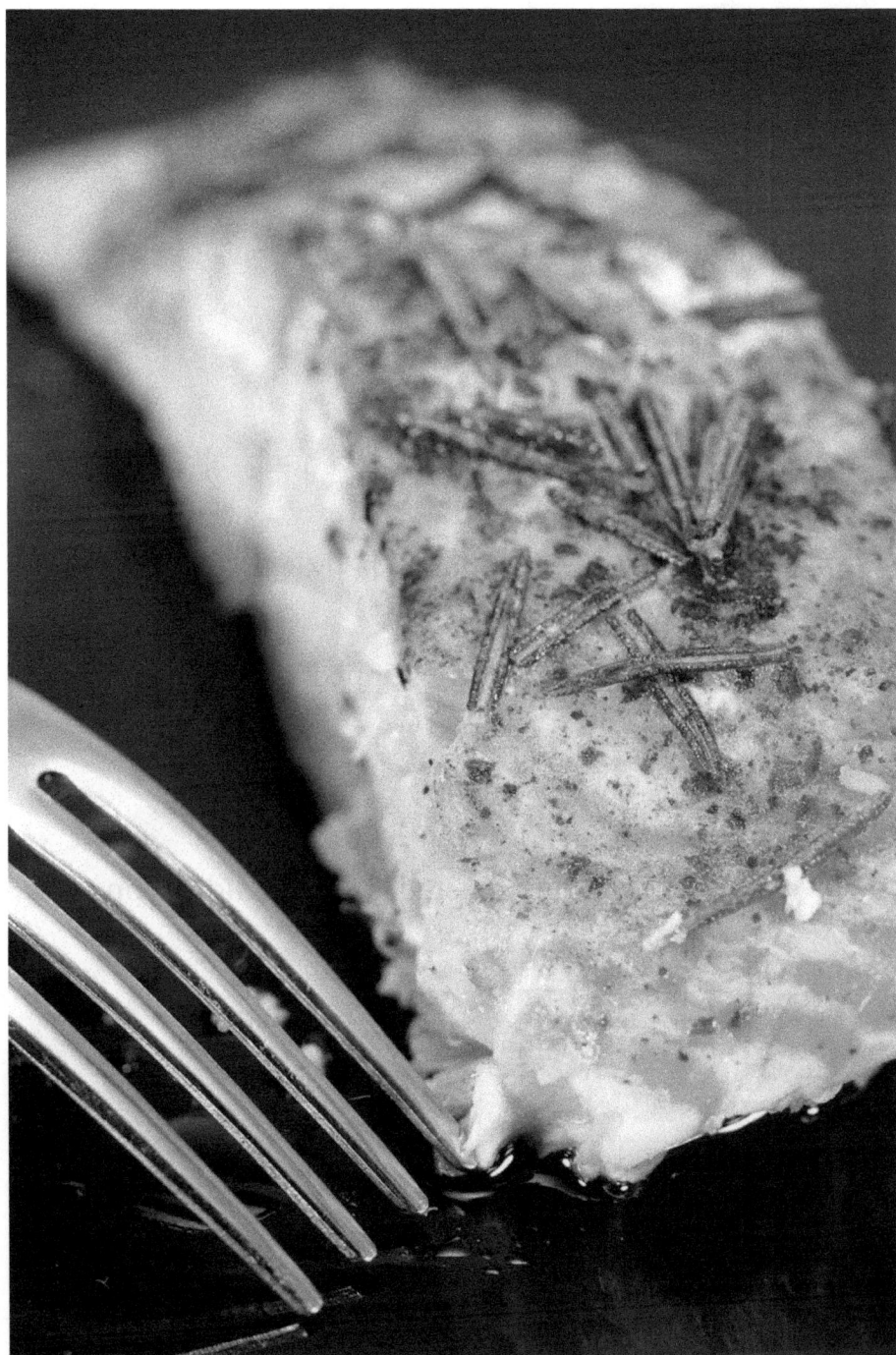

Easy Seafood French Stew

Servings: 12

Cooking Time: 45 Minutes

Ingredients:

- Pepper and Salt
- 1/2 lb. littleneck clams
- 1/2 lb. mussels
- 1 lb. shrimp, peeled and deveined
- 1 large lobster
- 2 lbs. assorted small whole fresh fish, scaled and cleaned
- 2 tbsp parsley, finely chopped
- 2 tbsp garlic, chopped
- 1 cup fennel, julienned
- Juice and zest of one orange
- 3 cups tomatoes, peeled, seeded, and chopped
- 1 cup leeks, julienned
- Pinch of Saffron
- 1 cup white wine
- Water
- 1 lb. fish bones
- 2 sprigs thyme
- 8 peppercorns
- 1 bay leaf
- 3 cloves garlic

- Salt and pepper
- 1/2 cup chopped celery
- 1/2 cup chopped onion
- 2 tbsp olive oil

Directions:

1. Do the stew: Heat oil in a large saucepan. Sauté the celery and onions for 3 minutes. Season with pepper and salt. Stir in the garlic and cook for about a minute. Add the thyme, peppercorns, and bay leaves. Stir in the wine, water and fish bones. Let it boil then before reducing to a simmer. Take the pan off the fire and strain broth into another container.

2. For the Bouillabaisse: Bring the strained broth to a simmer and stir in the parsley, leeks, orange juice, orange zest, garlic, fennel, tomatoes and saffron. Sprinkle with pepper and salt. Stir in the lobsters and fish. Let it simmer for eight minutes before stirring in the clams, mussels and shrimps. For six minutes, allow to cook while covered before seasoning again with pepper and salt.

3. Assemble in a shallow dish all the seafood and pour the broth over it.

Nutrition Info: Calories per serving: 348; Carbs: 20.0g; Protein: 31.8g; Fat: 15.2g

Lime Squid And Capers Mix

Servings: 6

Cooking Time: 20 Minutes

Ingredients:

- 1 pound baby squid, cleaned, body and tentacles chopped
- ½ teaspoon lime zest, grated
- 1 tablespoon lime juice
- ½ teaspoon orange zest, grated
- 3 tablespoons olive oil
- 1 teaspoon red pepper flakes, crushed
- 1 tablespoon parsley, chopped
- 4 garlic cloves, minced
- 1 shallot, chopped
- 2 tablespoons capers, drained
- 1 cup chicken stock
- 2 tablespoons red wine vinegar
- Salt and black pepper to the taste

Directions:

1. Heat up a pan with the oil over medium-high heat, add the lime zest, lime juice, orange zest and the rest of the ingredients except the squid and the parsley, stir, bring to a simmer and cook over medium heat for 10 minutes.

2. Add the remaining ingredients, stir, cook everything for 10 minutes more, divide into bowls and serve.

Nutrition Info: calories 302, fat 8.5, fiber 9.8, carbs 21.8, protein 11.3

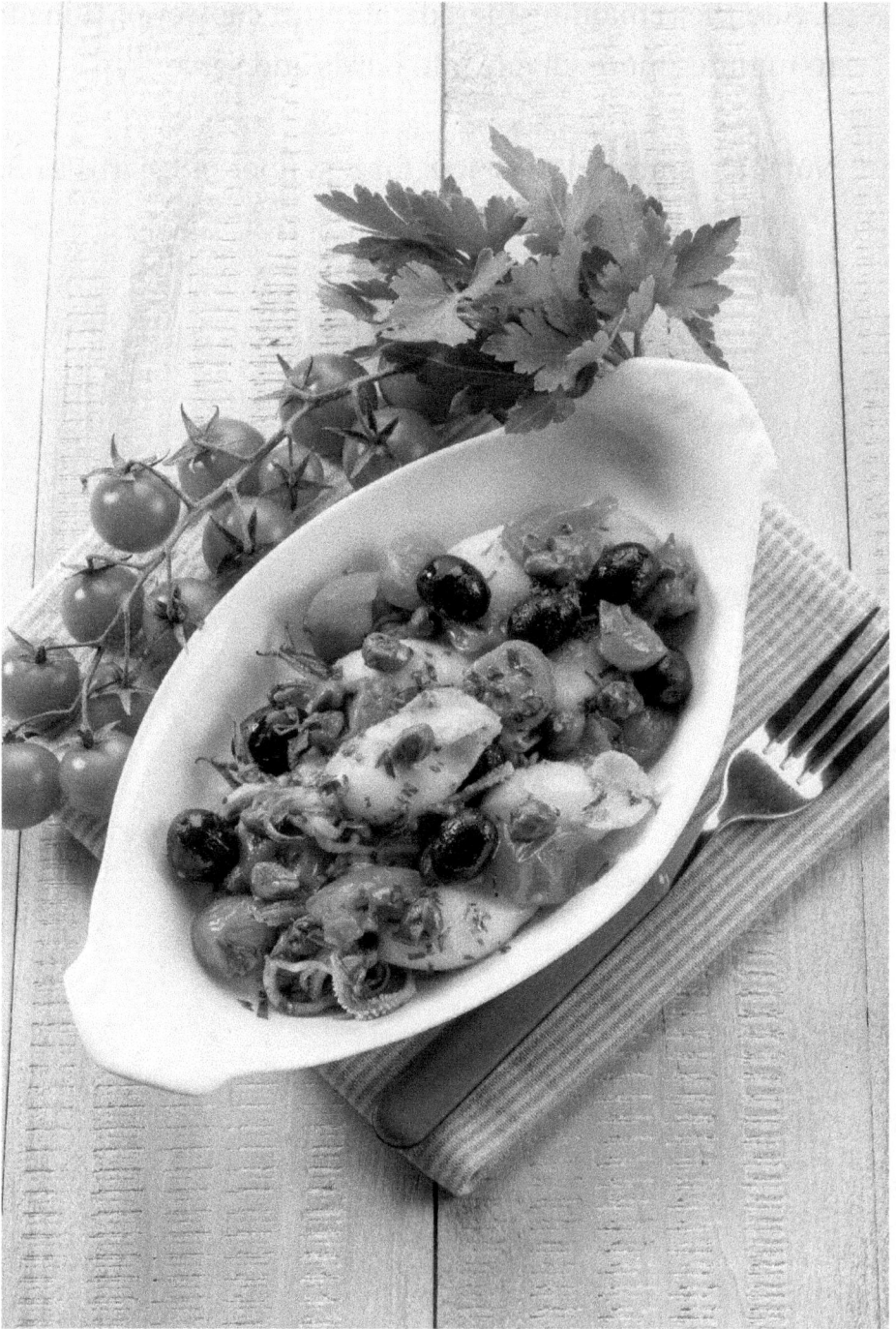

Salmon And Pineapple Sauce

Servings: 4

Cooking Time: 15 Minutes

Ingredients:
- 1 cup pineapple, chopped
- 14 oz salmon fillet
- ½ teaspoon salt
- ¾ teaspoon ground turmeric
- ¼ teaspoon cayenne pepper
- 1 teaspoon butter
- 1 teaspoon olive oil
- 1 tablespoon water
- ¼ teaspoon ground thyme
- ¼ cup of water

Directions:

1. Rub the salmon fillet with salt and ground turmeric.

2. Brush the fish with oil and grill in the grill for 3 minutes from each side at 385F.

3. Meanwhile, make the pineapple dip: blend the pineapple until smooth and transfer in the skillet.

4. Add water, butter, ground thyme, and cayenne pepper.

5. Brin the pineapple dip to boil and cook it without lid for 5 minutes over the high heat.

6. Cut the salmon fillet on 4 servings and arrange them in the serving plates.

7. Then top every salmon piece with pineapple dip.

Nutrition Info:Per Serving:calories 172, fat 8.4, fiber 0.7, carbs 5.8, protein 19.5

Wrapped Scallops

Servings: 12
Cooking Time: 6 Minutes

Ingredients:

- 12 medium scallops
- 12 thin bacon slices
- 2 teaspoons lemon juice
- 2 teaspoons olive oil
- A pinch of chili powder
- A pinch of cloves, ground
- Salt and black pepper to the taste

Directions:

1. Wrap each scallop in a bacon slice and secure with toothpicks.
2. Heat up a pan with the oil over medium-high heat, add the scallops and the rest of the ingredients, cook for 3 minutes on each side, divide between plates and serve.

Nutrition Info: calories 297, fat 24.3, fiber 9.6, carbs 22.4, protein 17.6

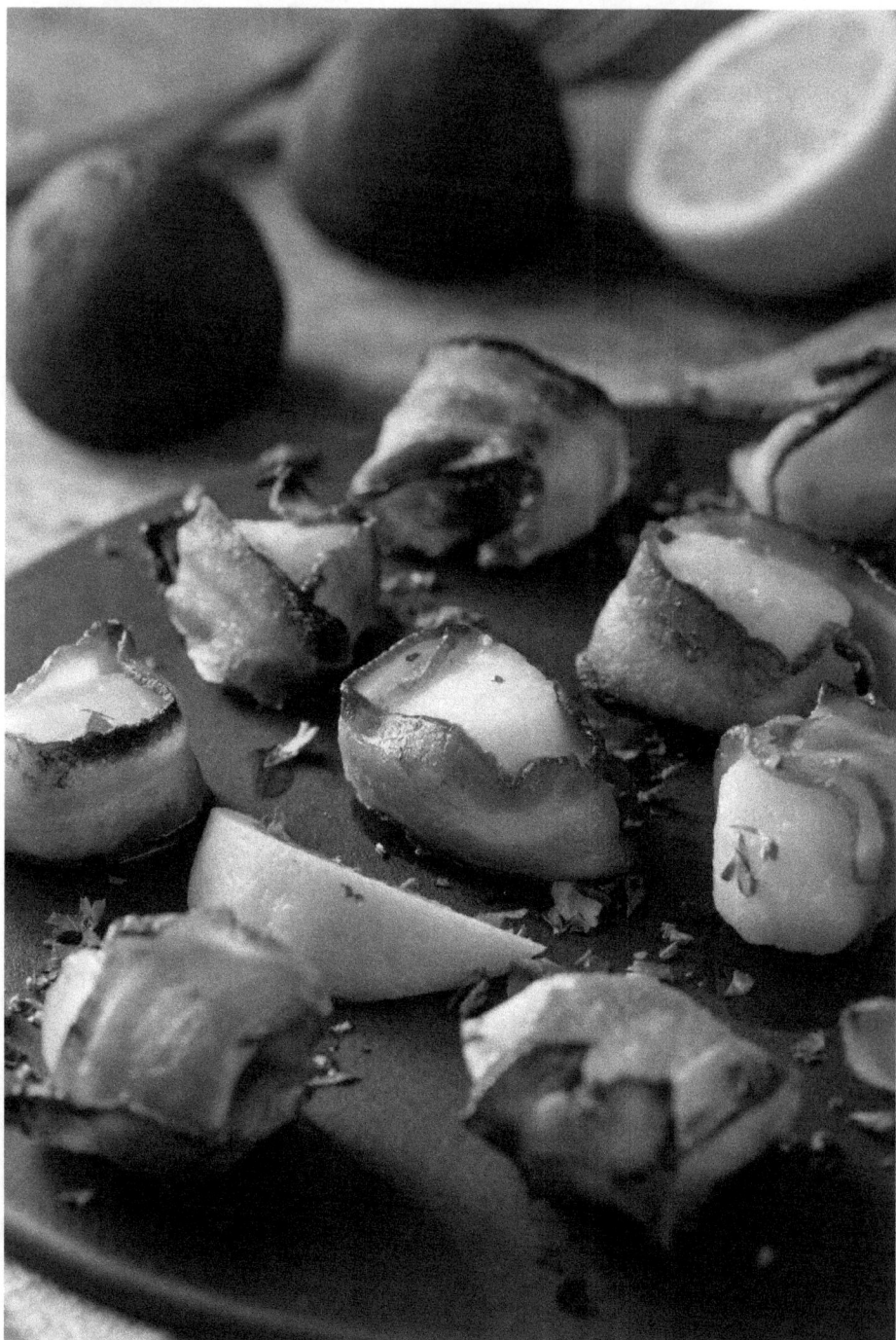

Walnut Salmon Mix

Servings: 4

Cooking Time: 25 Minutes

Ingredients:

- 12 oz salmon fillet
- 1/3 cup walnuts
- 1 tablespoon panko breadcrumbs
- 1 tablespoon dried oregano
- 1 tablespoon sunflower oil
- ½ teaspoon salt
- ½ teaspoon ground black pepper
- 1 tablespoon mustard

Directions:

1. Put the walnuts, panko bread crumbs, dried oregano, sunflower oil, salt, and ground black pepper in the blender.
2. Blend the ingredients until you get smooth and sticky mass.
3. After this, line the baking tray with baking paper.
4. Brush the salmon fillet with mustard from all sides and coat in the blended walnut mixture generously.
5. Bake the salmon for 25 minutes at 365F. Flip the salmon fillet on another side after 15 minutes of cooking.

Nutrition Info:Per Serving:calories 233, fat 15.9, fiber 1.9, carbs 4.7, protein 20.1

Pan Fried Tuna With Herbs And Nut

Servings: 4

Cooking Time: 5 Minutes

Ingredients:

- ¼ cup almonds, chopped finely
- ¼ cup fresh tangerine juice
- ½ tsp fennel seeds, chopped finely
- ½ tsp ground pepper, divided
- ½ tsp sea salt, divided
- 1 tbsp olive oil
- 2 tbsp. fresh mint, chopped finely
- 2 tbsp. red onion, chopped finely
- 4 pieces of 6-oz Tuna steak cut in half

Directions:

1. Mix fennel seeds, olive oil, mint, onion, tangerine juice and almonds in small bowl. Season with ¼ each of pepper and salt.

2. Season fish with the remaining pepper and salt.

3. On medium high fire, place a large nonstick fry pan and grease with cooking spray.

4. Pan fry tuna until desired doneness is reached or for one minute per side.

5. Transfer cooked tuna in serving plate, drizzle with dressing and serve.

Nutrition Info: Calories per Serving: 272; Fat: 9.7 g; Protein: 42 g; Carbohydrates: 4.2 g

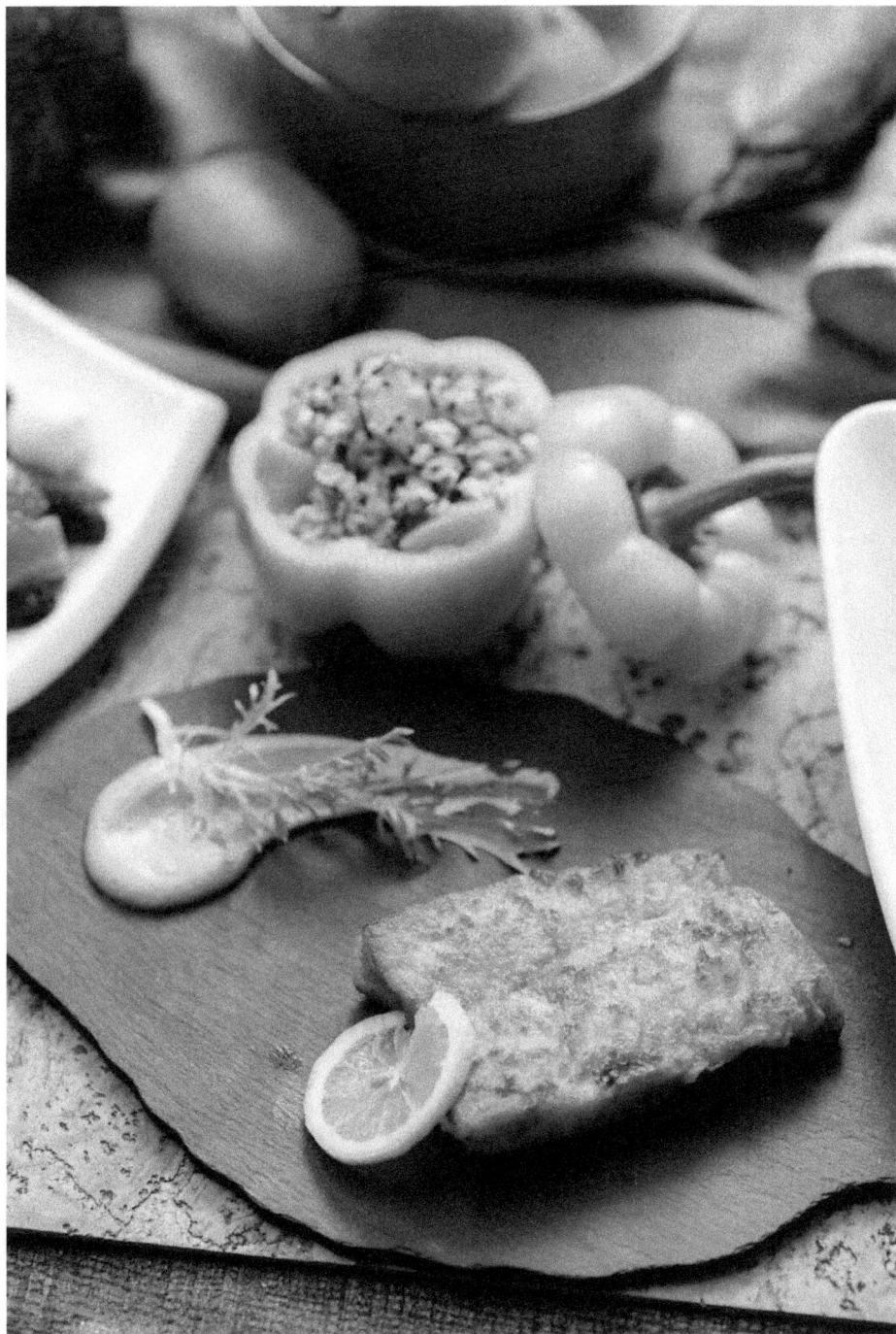

Tarragon Cod Fillets

Servings: 4

Cooking Time: 12 Minutes

Ingredients:

- 4 cod fillets, boneless
- ¼ cup capers, drained
- 1 tablespoon tarragon, chopped
- Sea salt and black pepper to the taste
- 2 tablespoons olive oil
- 2 tablespoons parsley, chopped
- 1 tablespoon olive oil
- 1 tablespoon lemon juice

Directions:

1. Heat up a pan with the oil over medium-high heat, add the fish and cook
for 3 minutes on each side.
2. Add the rest of the ingredients, cook everything for 7 minutes more, divide between plates and serve.

Nutrition Info: calories 162, fat 9.6, fiber 4.3, carbs 12.4, protein 16.5

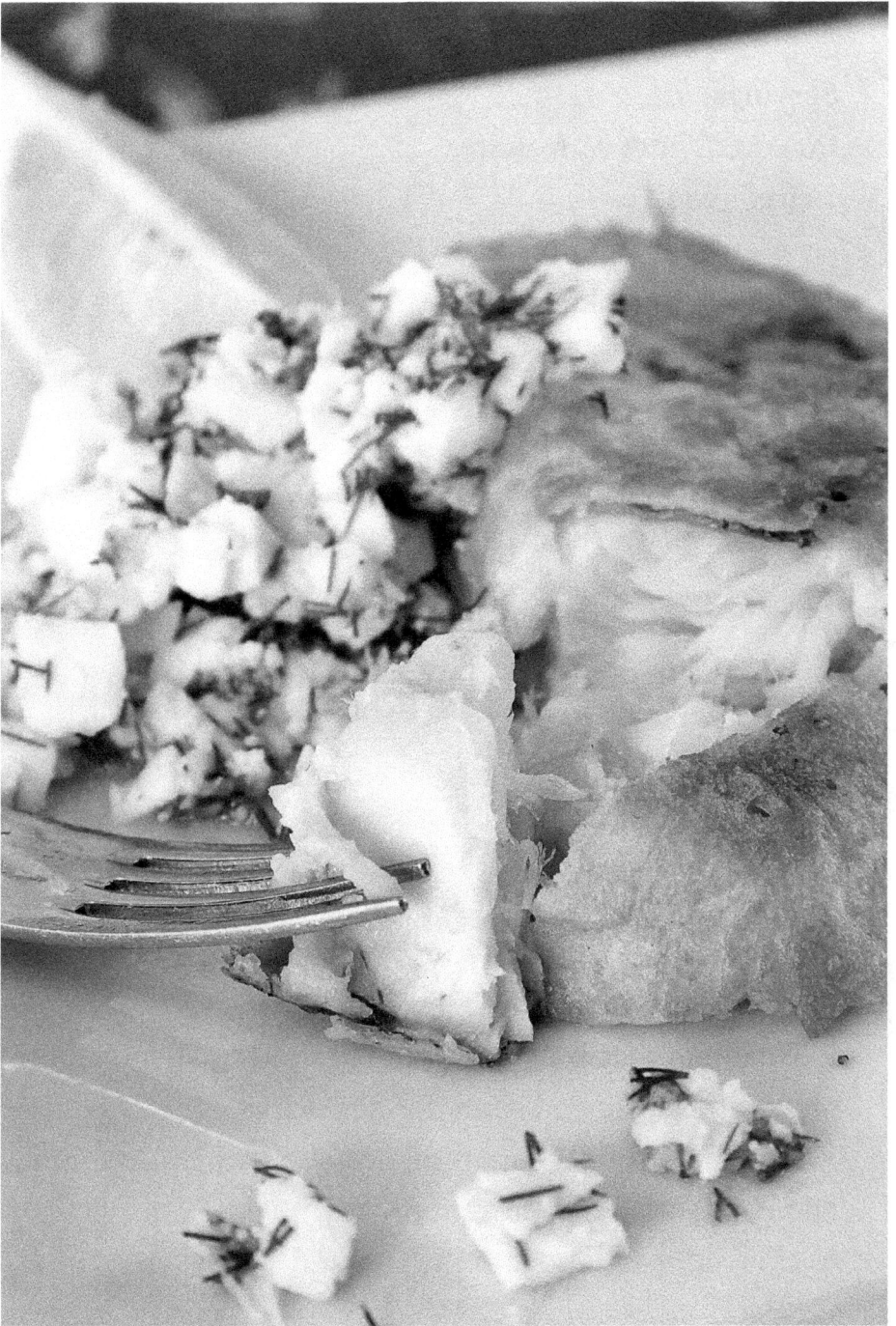

Cayenne Cod And Tomatoes

Servings: 4

Cooking Time: 25 Minutes

Ingredients:

- 1 teaspoon lime juice
- Salt and black pepper to the taste
- 1 teaspoon sweet paprika
- 1 teaspoon cayenne pepper
- 2 tablespoons olive oil
- 1 yellow onion, chopped
- 2 garlic cloves, minced
- 4 cod fillets, boneless
- A pinch of cloves, ground
- ½ cup chicken stock
- ½ pound cherry tomatoes, cubed

Directions:

1. Heat up a pan with the oil over medium-high heat add the cod, salt, pepper and the cayenne, cook for 4 minutes on each side and divide between plates.

2. Heat up the same pan over medium-high heat, add the onion and garlic and sauté for 5 minutes.

3. Add the rest of the ingredients, stir, bring to a simmer and cook for 10 minutes more.

4. Divide the mix next to the fish and serve.

Nutrition Info: calories 232, fat 16.5, fiber 11.1, carbs 24.8, protein 16.5

Cod And Mustard Sauce

Servings: 4

Cooking Time: 45 Minutes

Ingredients:

- 1-pound cod fillet
- 1 carrot, peeled
- 1 bell pepper, chopped
- 1 white onion, chopped
- 1 eggplant, peeled, chopped
- 2 tablespoons butter
- 1 tablespoon olive oil
- 1 teaspoon coriander seeds
- 1 teaspoon salt
- 1 teaspoon dried dill
- 1 teaspoon honey
- 1 tablespoon Mustard

Directions:

1. Chop the cod fillet roughly.
2. Line the baking tray with baking paper and arrange the fish in it.
3. After this, mix up together mustard, honey, dried dill, salt, coriander seeds, olive oil, and butter.
4. Chop the carrot roughly.

5. Put all vegetables in the baking tray and sprinkle with honey mixture.

6. Preheat the oven to 365F.

7. Bake the sheet-pan fish for 45 minutes.

8. When all the vegetables and fish are soft, the meal is cooked.

Nutrition Info:Per Serving:calories 257, fat 11.6, fiber 6, carbs 15.9, protein 25.1

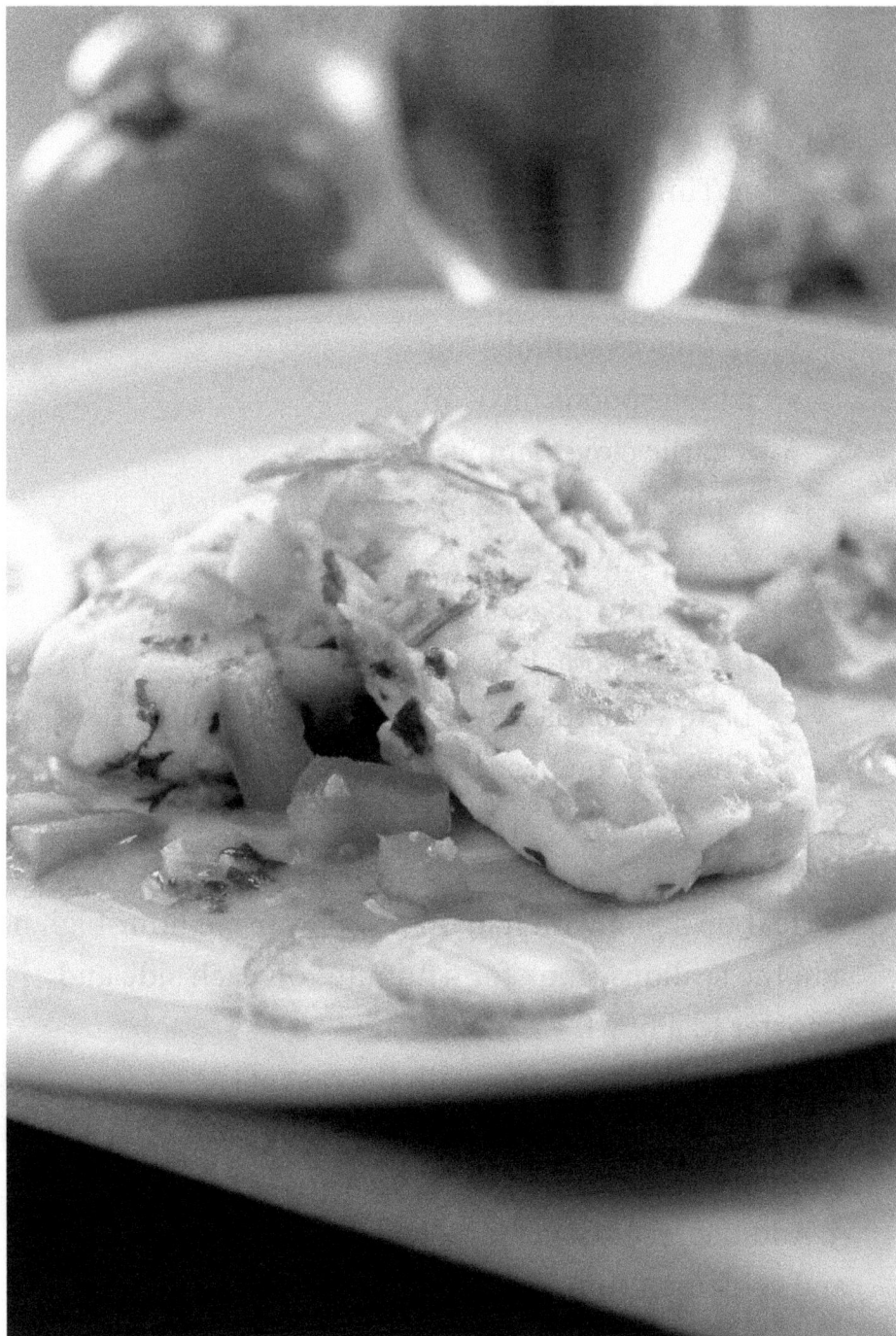

Garlic Scallops And Peas Mix

Servings: 6
Cooking Time: 20 Minutes

Ingredients:
- 12 ounces scallops
- 2 tablespoons olive oil
- 4 garlic cloves, minced
- A pinch of salt and black pepper
- ½ cup chicken stock
- 1 cup snow peas, sliced
- ½ tablespoon balsamic vinegar
- 1 cup scallions, sliced
- 1 tablespoon basil, chopped

Directions:
1. Heat up a pan with half of the oil over medium-high heat, add the scallops, cook for 5 minutes on each side and transfer to a bowl.
2. Heat up the pan again with the rest of the oil over medium heat, add the scallions and the garlic and sauté for 2 minutes.
3. Add the rest of the ingredients, stir, bring to a simmer and cook for 5 minutes more.

4. Add the scallops to the pan, cook everything for 3 minutes, divide into bowls and serve.

Nutrition Info: calories 296, fat 11.8, fiber 9.8, carbs 26.5, protein 20.5

Shrimp And Beans Salad

Servings: 4

Cooking Time: 4 Minutes

Ingredients:

- 1 pound shrimp, peeled and deveined
- 30 ounces canned cannellini beans, drained and rinsed
- 2 tablespoons olive oil
- 1 cup cherry tomatoes, halved
- 1 teaspoon lemon zest, grated
- ½ cup red onion, chopped
- 4 handfuls baby arugula
- A pinch of salt and black pepper
- For the dressing:
- 3 tablespoons red wine vinegar
- 2 garlic cloves, minced
- ½ cup olive oil

Directions:

1. Heat up a pan with 2 tablespoons oil over medium-high heat, add the shrimp and cook for 2 minutes on each side.
2. In a salad bowl, combine the shrimp with the beans and the rest of the ingredients except the ones for the dressing and toss.

3. In a separate bowl, combine the vinegar with ½ cup oil and the garlic and whisk well.

4. Pour over the salad, toss and serve right away.

Nutrition Info: calories 207, fat 12.3, fiber 6.6, carbs 15.4, protein 8.7

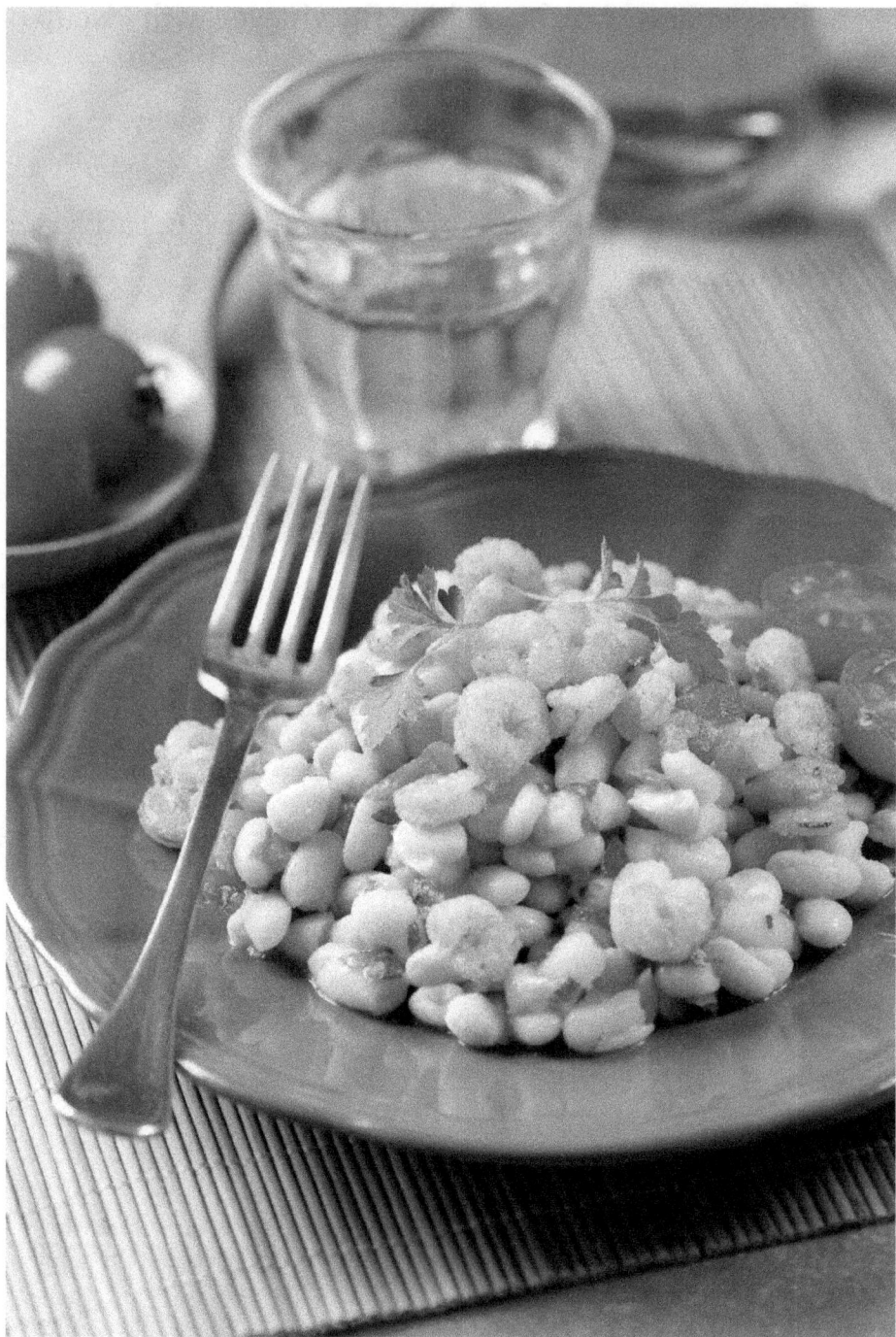

Lemony Prawns

Servings: 2

Cooking Time: 3 Minutes

Ingredients:
- 1/2 lb prawns
- 1/2 cup fish stock
- 1 tbsp fresh lemon juice
- 1 tbsp lemon zest, grated
- 1 tbsp olive oil
- 1 tbsp garlic, minced
- Pepper
- Salt

Directions:

1. Add all ingredients into the inner pot of instant pot and stir well.

2. Seal pot with lid and cook on high for 3 minutes.

3. Once done, release pressure using quick release. Remove lid.

4. Drain prawns and serve.

Nutrition Info: Calories 215 Fat 9.5 g Carbohydrates 3.9 g Sugar 0.4 g Protein 27.6 g Cholesterol 239 mg

Pesto And Lemon Halibut

Servings: 4
Cooking Time: 10 Minutes

Ingredients:
- 1 tbsp fresh lemon juice
- 1 tbsp lemon rind, grated
- 2 garlic cloves, peeled
- 2 tbsp olive oil
- ¼ cup Parmesan Cheese, freshly grated
- 2/3 cups firmly packed basil leaves
- 1/8 tsp freshly ground black pepper
- ¼ tsp salt, divided
- 4 pcs 6-oz halibut fillets

Directions:
1. Preheat grill to medium fire and grease grate with cooking spray.
2. Season fillets with pepper and 1/8 tsp salt. Place on grill and cook until halibut is flaky around 4 minutes per side.
3. Meanwhile, make your lemon pesto by combining lemon juice, lemon rind, garlic, olive oil, Parmesan cheese, basil leaves and remaining salt in a blender. Pulse mixture until finely minced but not pureed.

4. Once fish is done cooking, transfer to a serving platter, pour over the lemon pesto sauce, serve and enjoy.

Nutrition Info: Calories per Serving: 277.4; Fat: 13g; Protein: 38.7g; Carbs: 1.4g

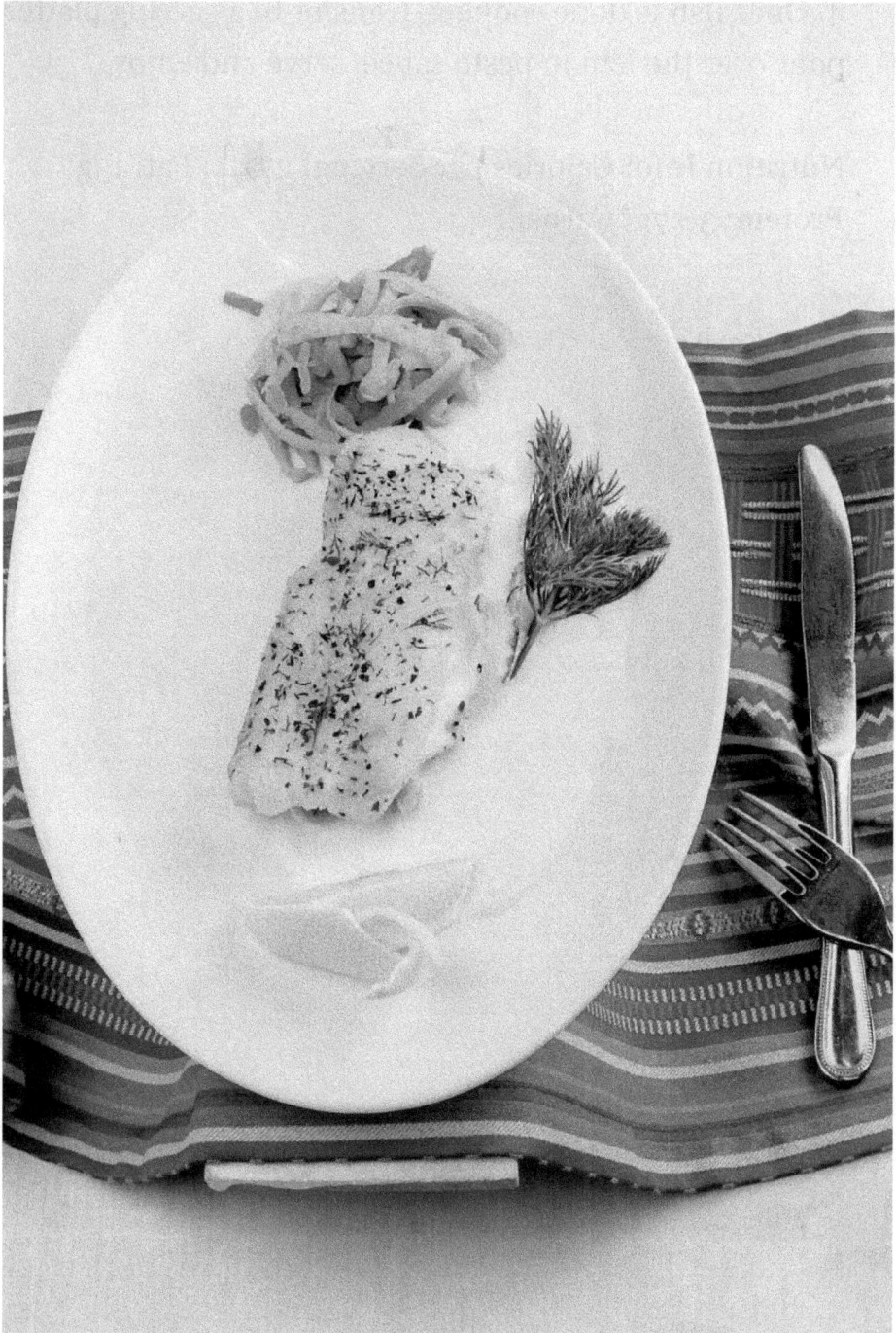

Stuffed Branzino

Servings: 7
Cooking Time: 40 Minutes

Ingredients:

- 6 oz fennel bulb, trimmed
- 1 teaspoon ground coriander
- ½ teaspoon ground black pepper
- 1 tablespoon lemon juice
- 1 teaspoon salt
- 1 teaspoon dried oregano
- 1 teaspoon dried cilantro
- 1 tablespoon butter, unsalted
- 1.5-pound whole branzino, trimmed, peeled
- 1 tablespoon sunflower oil

Directions:
1. Slice fennel bulb.
2. Rub the branzino with ground coriander, black pepper, salt, oregano, and cilantro.
3. Then sprinkle it with lemon juice and sunflower oil.
4. After this, fill the branzino with butter and sliced fennel and wrap the fish in the foil.
5. Bake the fish for 40 minutes at 365F.

6. Then discard the foil from the fish and cut it on the servings.

Nutrition Info:Per Serving:calories 245, fat 8.4, fiber 0.9, carbs 2.1, protein 39.2

Tomato Olive Fish Fillets

Servings: 4

Cooking Time: 8 Minutes

Ingredients:
- 2 lbs halibut fish fillets
- 2 oregano sprigs
- 2 rosemary sprigs
- 2 tbsp fresh lime juice
- 1 cup olives, pitted
- 28 oz can tomatoes, diced
- 1 tbsp garlic, minced
- 1 onion, chopped
- 2 tbsp olive oil

Directions:

1. Add oil into the inner pot of instant pot and set the pot on sauté mode.

2. Add onion and sauté for 3 minutes.

3. Add garlic and sauté for a minute.

4. Add lime juice, olives, herb sprigs, and tomatoes and stir well.

5. Seal pot with lid and cook on high for 3 minutes.

6. Once done, release pressure using quick release. Remove lid.

7. Add fish fillets and seal pot again with lid and cook on high for 2 minutes.

8. Once done, release pressure using quick release. Remove lid. 9. Serve and enjoy.

Nutrition Info: Calories 333 Fat 19.1 g Carbohydrates 31.8 g Sugar 8.4 g Protein 13.4 g Cholesterol 5 mg

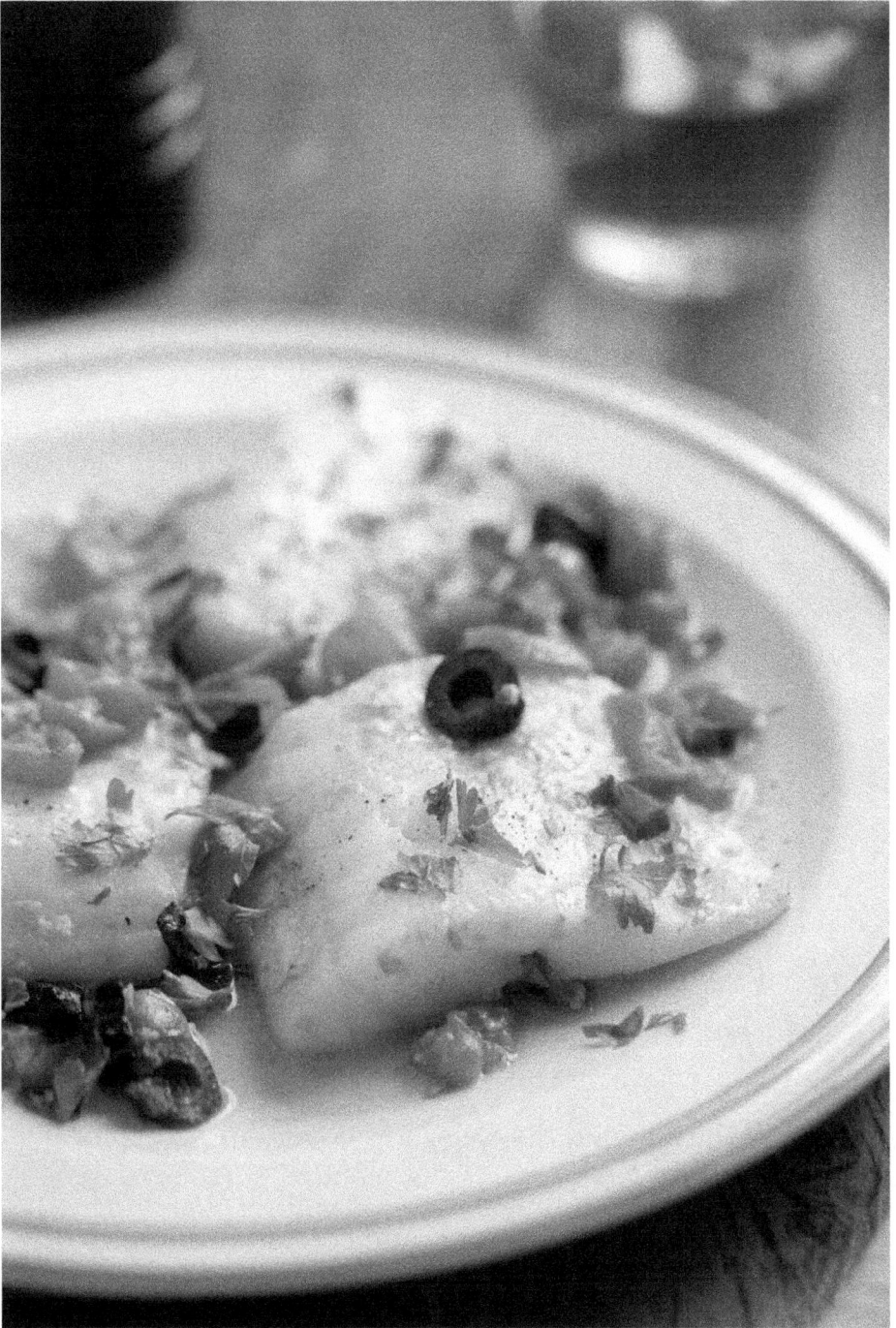

Steamed Mussels Thai Style

Servings: 4

Cooking Time: 15 Minutes

Ingredients:
- ¼ cup minced shallots
- ½ tsp Madras curry
- 1 cup dry white wine
- 1 small bay leaf
- 1 tbsp chopped fresh basil
- 1 tbsp chopped fresh cilantro
- 1 tbsp chopped fresh mint
- 2 lbs. mussel, cleaned and debearded
- 2 tbsp butter
- 4 medium garlic cloves, minced

Directions:

1. In a large heavy bottomed pot, on medium high fire add to pot the curry powder, bay leaf, wine plus the minced garlic and shallots. Bring to a boil and simmer for 3 minutes.

2. Add the cleaned mussels, stir, cover, and cook for 3 minutes.

3. Stir mussels again, cover, and cook for another 2 or 3 minutes. Cooking is done when majority of shells have opened.

4. With a slotted spoon, transfer cooked mussels in a large bowl. Discard any unopened mussels.

5. Continue heating pot with sauce. Add butter and the chopped herbs.

6. Season with pepper and salt to taste.

7. Once good, pour over mussels, serve and enjoy.

Nutrition Info: Calories per Serving: 407.2; Protein: 43.4g; Fat: 21.2g; Carbs: 10.8g

Oregano Citrus Salmon

Servings: 2

Cooking Time: 15 Minutes

Ingredients:
- 2 salmon fillets (5 oz each fish fillet)
- ½ teaspoon garlic powder
- ¾ teaspoon chili flakes
- ¾ teaspoon ground coriander
- ½ teaspoon salt
- 1 tablespoon butter
- ½ teaspoon dried oregano
- 1 orange, peel

Directions:

1. In the shallow bowl make the spice mix from garlic powder, chili flakes, ground coriander, salt, and dried oregano.

2. Then coat the salmon fillets in the spice mix.

3. Slice the orange and place it in the skillet.

4. Add butter and roast the sliced orange until the butter is melted.

5. Then remove the sliced orange from the skillet.

6. Add salmon fillets and roast them for 4 minutes from each side over the medium heat.

7. After this, top the salmon with roasted sliced orange and close the lid. 8. Cook the fish for 5 minutes more over the low heat.

Nutrition Info:Per Serving:calories 285, fat 14.7, fiber 2.5, carbs 11.6, protein 28.6

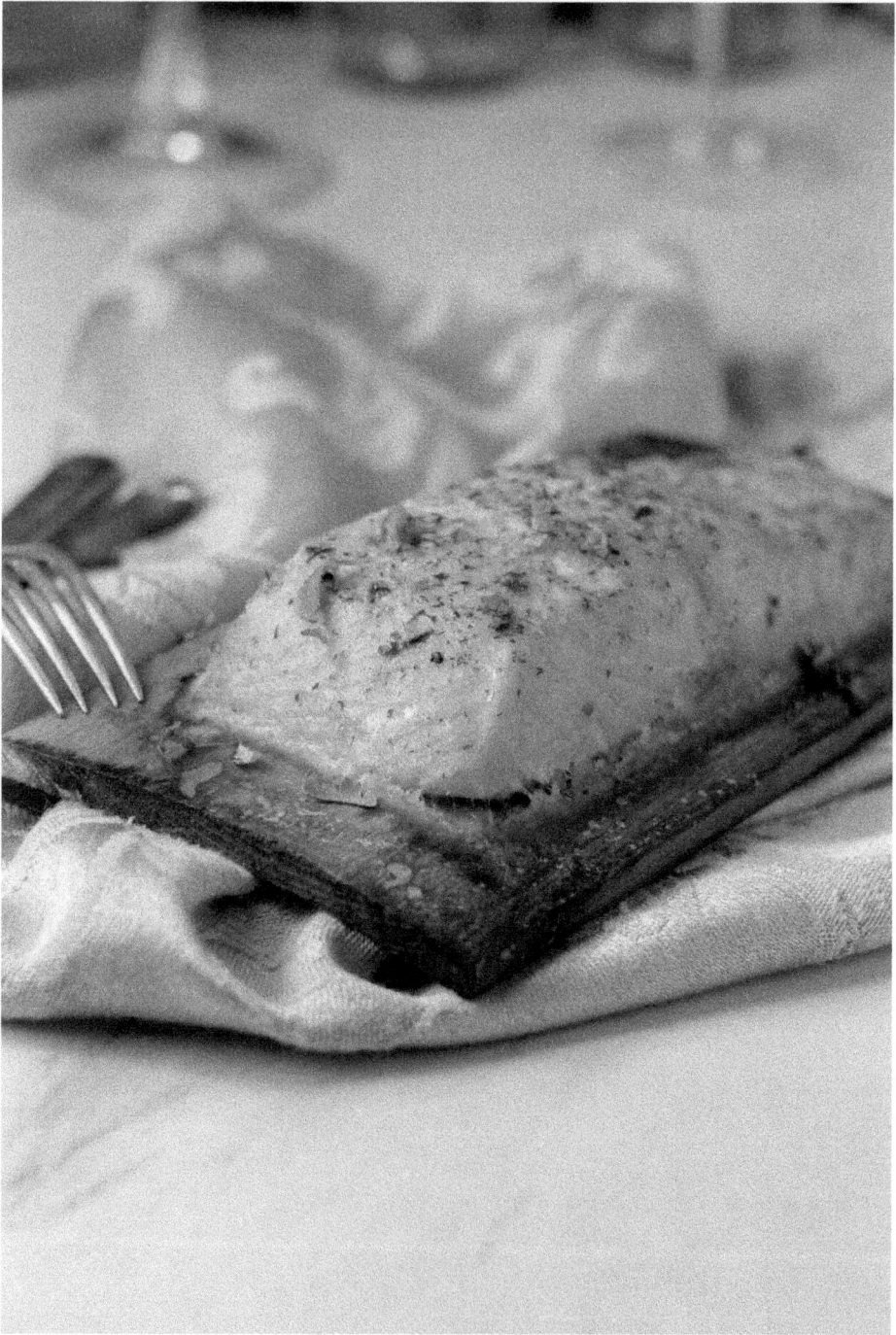

Nutmeg Sea Bass

Servings: 4

Cooking Time: 10 Minutes

Ingredients:

- 1 teaspoon fresh ginger, minced
- 10 oz sea bass fillet (4 fillets)
- 1 tablespoon butter
- 1 teaspoon minced garlic
- ¼ teaspoon ground nutmeg
- ½ teaspoon salt

Directions:

1. Toss butter in the skillet and melt it.
2. Add minced garlic, ground nutmeg, salt, and fresh ginger.
3. Roast the mixture for 1 minute.
4. Then add seabass fillet.
5. Fryt the fish for 3 minutes from each side.

Nutrition Info:Per Serving:calories 205, fat 13.5, fiber 0.8, carbs 0.6, protein 19.7

Shrimp Kebabs

Servings: 2

Cooking Time: 5 Minutes

Ingredients:

- 4 King prawns, peeled
- 1 tablespoon lemon juice
- ¾ teaspoon ground coriander
- ½ teaspoon salt
- 1 tablespoon tomato sauce
- 1 tablespoon olive oil

Directions:

1. Skew the shrimps on the skewers and sprinkle them with lemon juice, ground coriander, salt, and tomato sauce.
2. Then drizzle the shrimps with olive oil.
3. Preheat grill to 385F.
4. Grill the shrimp kebabs for 2 minutes from each side.

Nutrition Info:Per Serving:calories 106, fat 7.5, fiber 0.4, carbs 0.6, protein 9.1

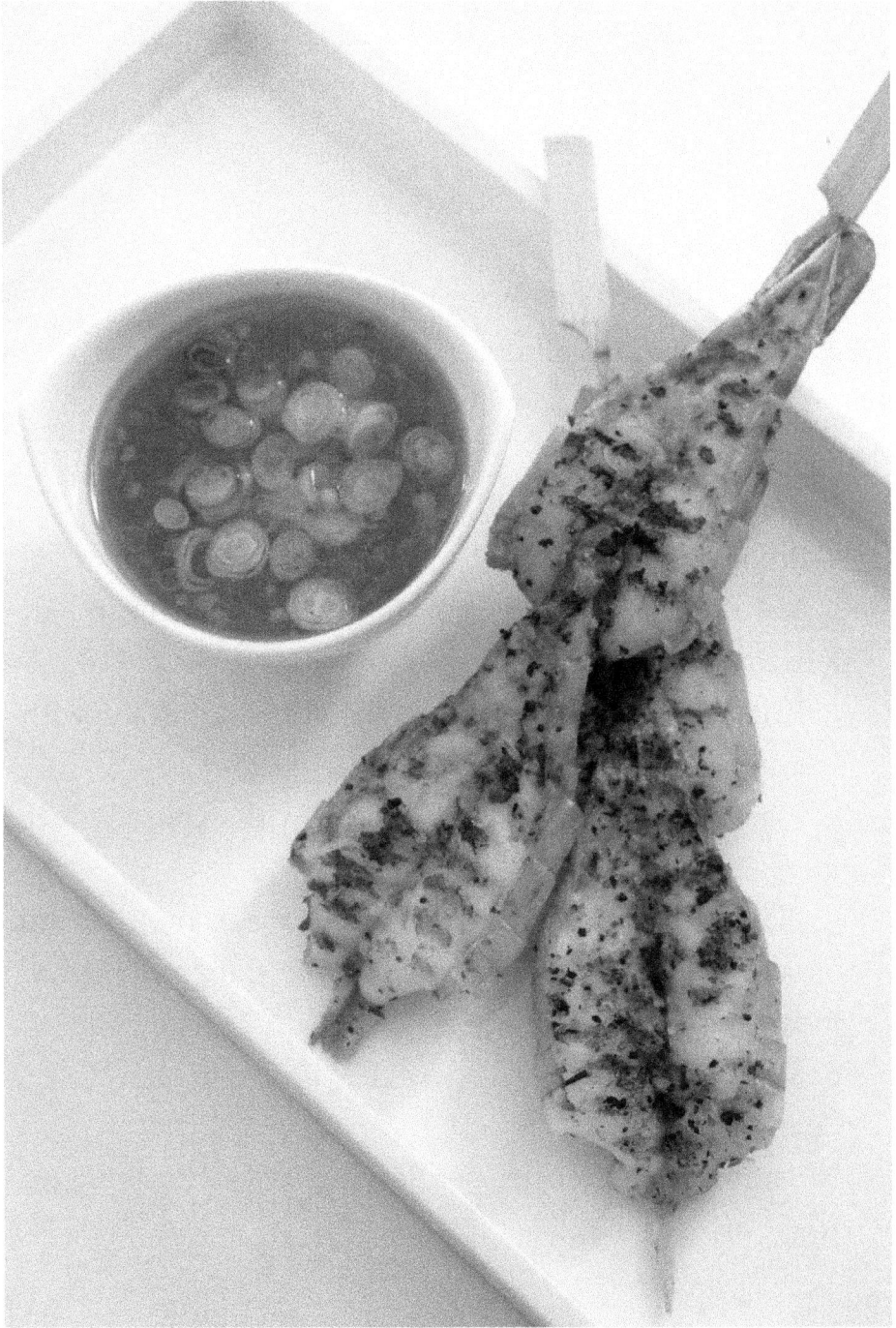

Easy Broiled Lobster Tails

Servings: 2

Cooking Time: 10 Minutes

Ingredients:

- 1 6-oz frozen lobster tails
- 1 tbsp olive oil
- 1 tsp lemon pepper seasoning

Directions:

1. Preheat oven broiler.
2. With kitchen scissors, cut thawed lobster tails in half lengthwise.
3. Brush with oil the exposed lobster meat. Season with lemon pepper.
4. Place lobster tails in baking sheet with exposed meat facing up.
5. Place on top broiler rack and broil for 10 minutes until lobster meat is lightly browned on the sides and center meat is opaque.
6. Serve and enjoy.

Nutrition Info: Calories per Serving: 175.6; Protein: 3g; Fat: 10g; Carbs: 18.4g

Cajun Garlic Shrimp Noodle Bowl

Servings: 2

Cooking Time: 15 Minutes

Ingredients:

- ½ teaspoon salt
- 1 onion, sliced
- 1 red pepper, sliced
- 1 tablespoon butter
- 1 teaspoon garlic granules
- 1 teaspoon onion powder
- 1 teaspoon paprika
- 2 large zucchinis, cut into noodle strips
- 20 jumbo shrimps, shells removed and deveined
- 3 cloves garlic, minced
- 3 tablespoon ghee
- A dash of cayenne pepper
- A dash of red pepper flakes

Directions:

1. Prepare the Cajun seasoning by mixing the onion powder, garlic granules, pepper flakes, cayenne pepper, paprika and salt. Toss in the shrimp to coat in the seasoning.

2. In a skillet, heat the ghee and sauté the garlic. Add in the red pepper and onions and continue sautéing for 4 minutes.

3. Add the Cajun shrimp and cook until opaque. Set aside.

4. In another pan, heat the butter and sauté the zucchini noodles for three minutes.

5. Assemble by the placing the Cajun shrimps on top of the zucchini
noodles.

Nutrition Info: Calories per Serving: 712; Fat: 30.0g; Protein: 97.8g; Carbs: 20.2g

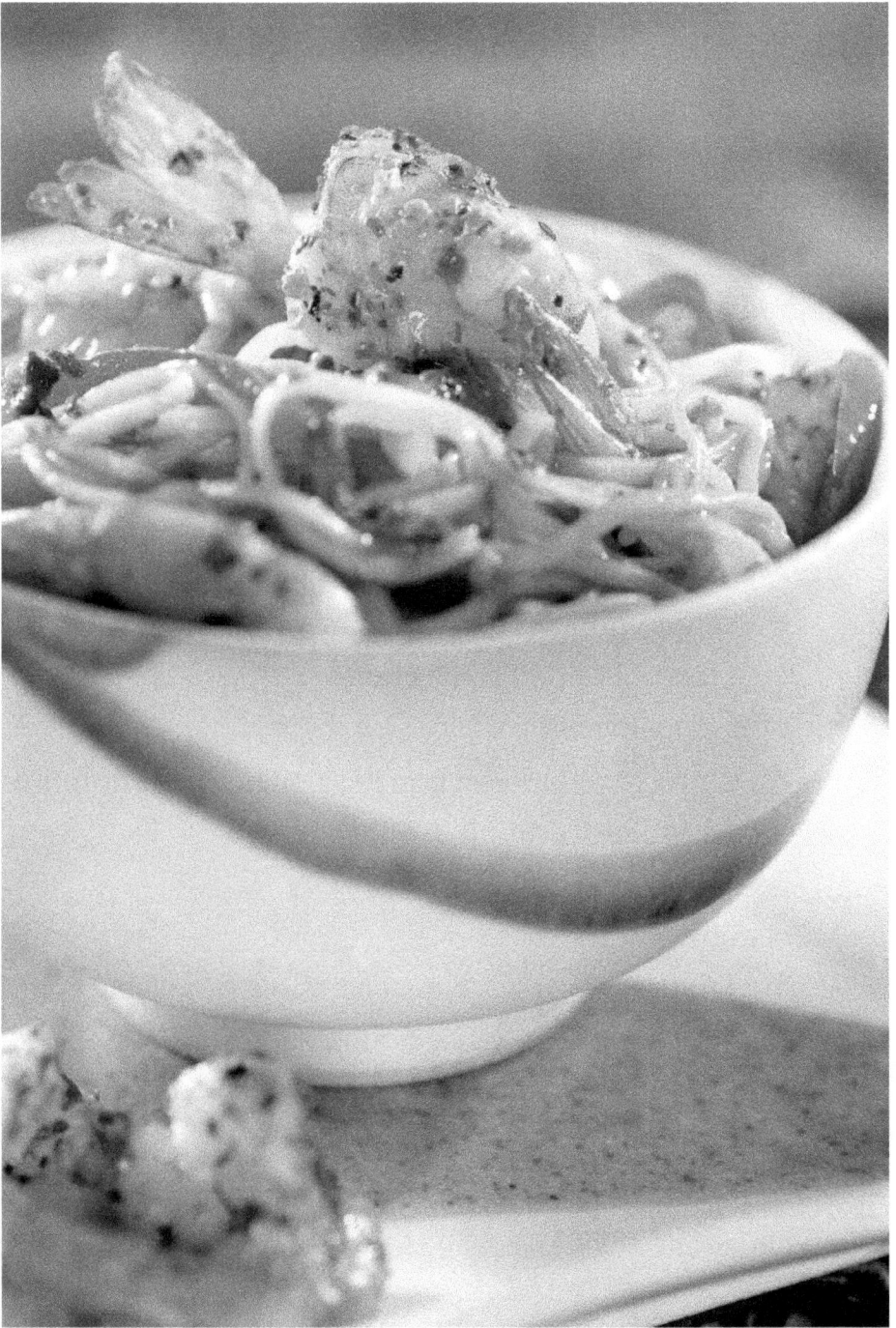

Red Peppers & Pineapple Topped Mahi-mahi

Servings: 4

Cooking Time: 30 Minutes

Ingredients:

- ¼ tsp black pepper
- ¼ tsp salt
- 1 cup whole wheat couscous
- 1 red bell pepper, diced
- 2 1/3 cups low sodium chicken broth
- 2 cups chopped fresh pineapple
- 2 tbsp. chopped fresh chives
- 2 tsp. olive oil
- 4 pieces of skinless, boneless mahi mahi (dolphin fish) fillets (around 4-oz each)

Directions:

1. On high fire, add 1 1/3 cups broth to a small saucepan and heat until boiling. Once boiling, add couscous. Turn off fire, cover and set aside to allow liquid to be fully absorbed around 5 minutes.

2. On medium high fire, place a large nonstick saucepan and heat oil.

3. Season fish on both sides with pepper and salt. Add mahi mahi to hot pan and pan fry until golden around one minute each side. Once cooked, transfer to plate.

4. On same pan, sauté bell pepper and pineapples until soft, around 2 minutes on medium high fire.

5. Add couscous to pan along with chives, and remaining broth.

6. On top of the mixture in pan, place fish. With foil, cover pan and continue cooking until fish is steaming and tender underneath the foil, around 3-5 minutes.

Nutrition Info: Calories per serving: 302; Protein: 43.1g; Fat: 4.8g; Carbs: 22.0g

Kale, Beets And Cod Mix

Servings: 4

Cooking Time: 20 Minutes

Ingredients:

- 2 tablespoons apple cider vinegar
- ½ cup chicken stock
- 1 red onion, sliced
- 4 golden beets, trimmed, peeled and cubed
- 2 tablespoons olive oil
- Salt and black pepper to the taste
- 4 cups kale, torn
- 2 tablespoons walnuts, chopped
- 1 pound cod fillets, boneless, skinless and cubed

Directions:

1. Heat up a pan with the oil over medium-high heat, add the onion and the beets and cook for 3-4 minutes.
2. Add the rest of the ingredients except the fish and the walnuts, stir, bring to a simmer and cook for 5 minutes more.
3. Add the fish, cook for 10 minutes, divide between plates and serve.

Nutrition Info: calories 285, fat 7.6, fiber 6.5, carbs 16.7, protein 12.5

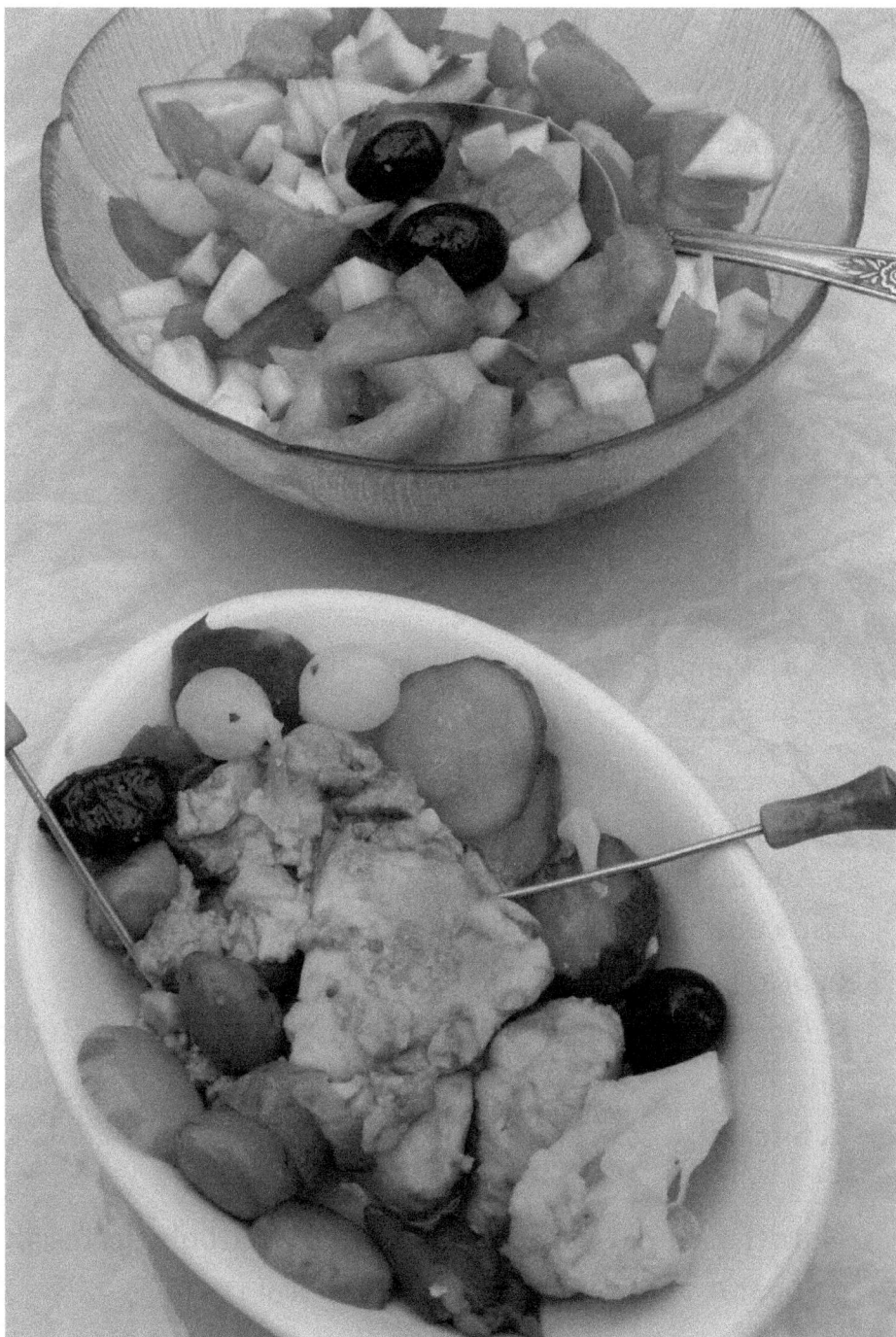

Shrimp Scampi

Servings: 6
Cooking Time: 8 Minutes

Ingredients:
- 1 lb whole wheat penne pasta
- 1 lb frozen shrimp
- 2 tbsp garlic, minced
- 1/4 tsp cayenne
- 1/2 tbsp Italian seasoning
- 1/4 cup olive oil
- 3 1/2 cups fish stock
- Pepper
- Salt

Directions:
1. Add all ingredients into the inner pot of instant pot and stir well.
2. Seal pot with lid and cook on high for 6 minutes.
3. Once done, release pressure using quick release. Remove lid.
4. Stir well and serve.

Nutrition Info: Calories 435 Fat 12.6 g Carbohydrates 54.9 g Sugar 0.1 g Protein 30.6 g Cholesterol 116 mg

Orange Rosemary Seared Salmon

Servings: 4

Cooking Time: 10 Minutes

Ingredients:

- ½ cup chicken stock
- 1 cup fresh orange juice
- 1 tablespoon coconut oil
- 1 tablespoon tapioca starch
- 2 garlic cloves, minced
- 2 tablespoon fresh lemon juice
- 2 teaspoon fresh rosemary, minced
- 2 teaspoon orange zest
- 4 salmon fillets, skins removed
- Salt and pepper to taste

Directions:

1. Season the salmon fillet on both sides.

2. In a skillet, heat coconut oil over medium high heat. Cook the salmon fillets for 5 minutes on each side. Set aside.

3. In a mixing bowl, combine the orange juice, chicken stock, lemon juice and orange zest.

4. In the skillet, sauté the garlic and rosemary for 2 minutes and pour the orange juice mixture. Bring to a boil. Lower

the heat to medium low and simmer. Season with salt and pepper to taste.

5. Pour the sauce all over the salmon fillet then serve.

Nutrition Info: Calories per Serving: 493; Fat: 17.9g; Protein: 66.7g; Carbs: 12.8g

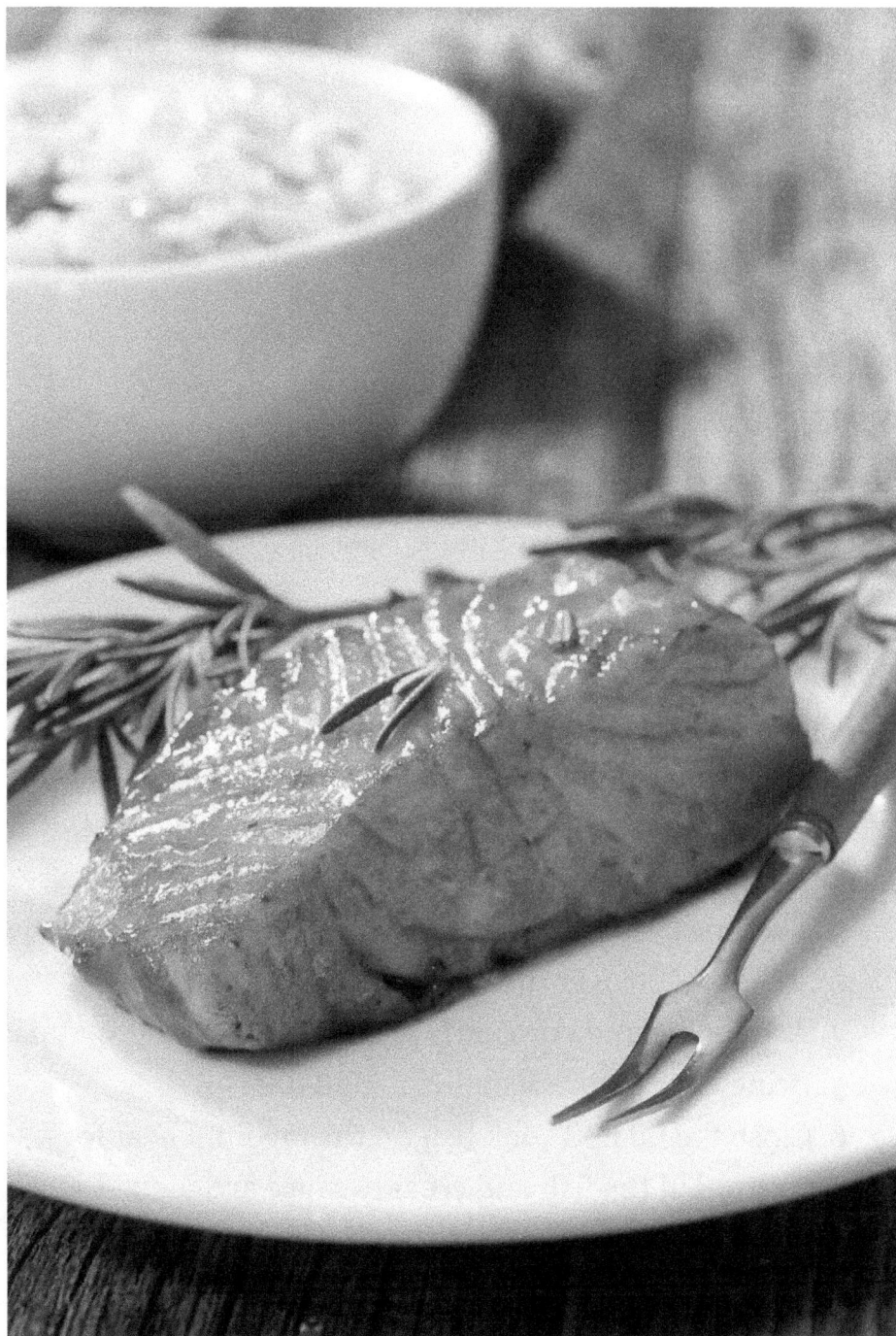

Dill Halibut

Servings: 3

Cooking Time: 10 Minutes

Ingredients:

- 13 oz halibut fillet
- 1/3 cup cream
- ¼ cup dill, chopped
- ½ teaspoon garlic powder
- ¼ teaspoon turmeric
- ¼ teaspoon ground paprika
- 1 teaspoon salt
- 1 teaspoon olive oil

Directions:

1. Chop the fish fillet on the big cubes and sprinkle them with garlic powder, turmeric, ground paprika, and salt.

2. Pour olive oil in the skillet and preheat it well.

3. Then place fish in the hot oil and roast it for 2 minutes from each side over the medium heat.

4. Add cream and stir gently with the help of the spatula.

5. Bring the mixture to boil and add dill.

6. Close the lid and cook fish on the medium heat for 5 minutes. Till the fish and creamy sauce are cooked.

7. Serve the halibut cubes with creamy sauce.

Nutrition Info:Per Serving:calories 170, fat 5.9, fiber 0.7, carbs 3.6, protein 25.1

Salmon And Mango Mix

Servings: 2

Cooking Time: 25 Minutes

Ingredients:
- 2 salmon fillets, skinless and boneless
- Salt and pepper to the taste
- 2 tablespoons olive oil
- 2 garlic cloves, minced
- 2 mangos, peeled and cubed
- 1 red chili, chopped
- 1 small piece ginger, grated
- Juice of 1 lime
- 1 tablespoon cilantro, chopped

Directions:

1. In a roasting pan, combine the salmon with the oil, garlic and the rest of the ingredients except the cilantro, toss, introduce in the oven at 350 degrees F and bake for 25 minutes.

2. Divide everything between plates and serve with the cilantro sprinkled on top.

Nutrition Info: calories 251, fat 15.9, fiber 5.9, carbs 26.4, protein 12.4

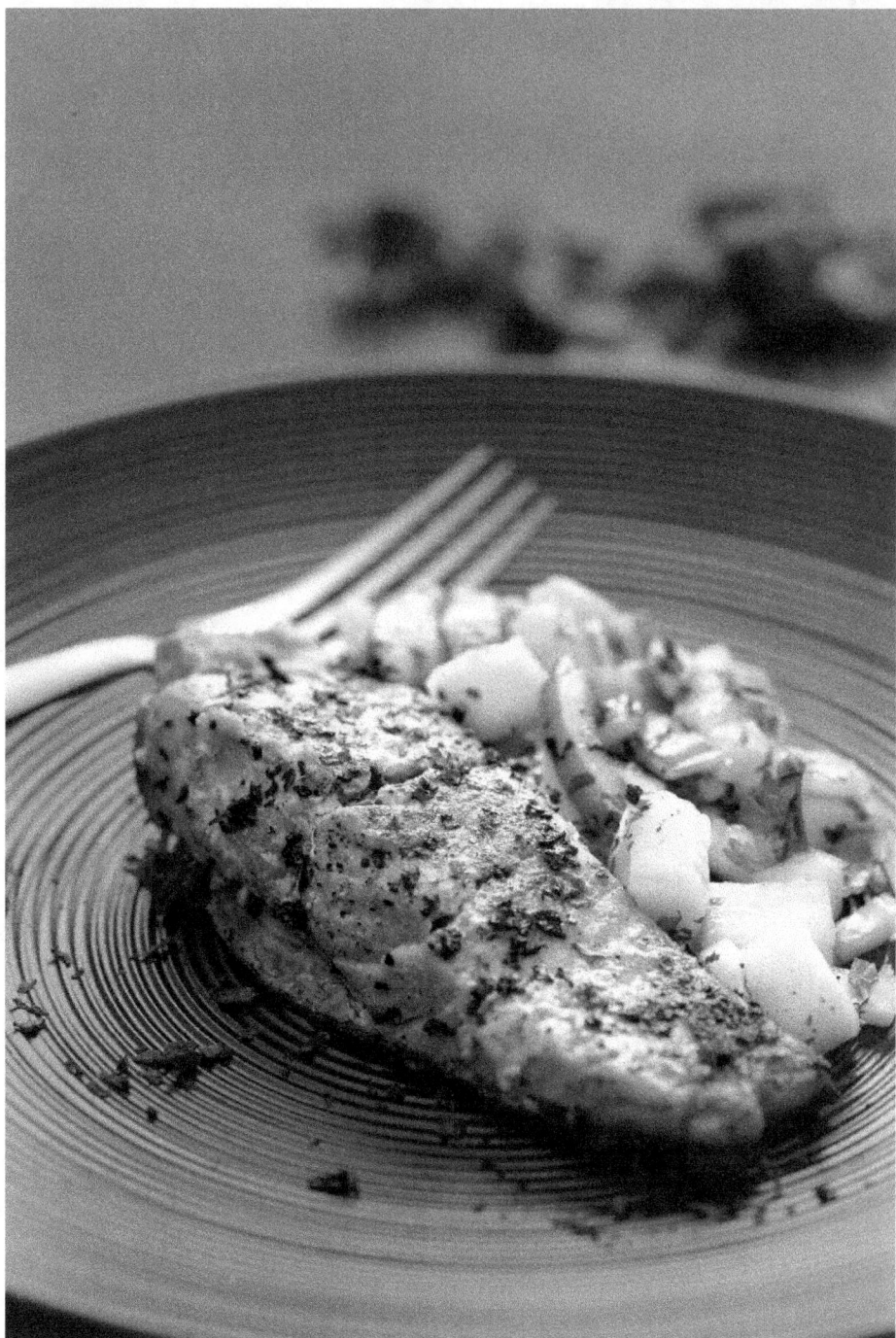

Delicious Shrimp Alfredo

Servings: 4
Cooking Time: 3 Minutes

Ingredients:
12 shrimp, remove shells
1 tbsp garlic, minced
1/4 cup parmesan cheese
2 cups whole wheat rotini noodles
1 cup fish broth
15 oz alfredo sauce
1 onion, chopped
Salt

Directions:
1. Add all ingredients except parmesan cheese into the instant pot and stir well.
2. Seal pot with lid and cook on high for 3 minutes.
3. Once done, release pressure using quick release. Remove lid.
4. Stir in cheese and serve.

Nutrition Info: Calories 669 Fat 23.1 g Carbohydrates 76 g Sugar 2.4 g Protein 37.8 g Cholesterol 190 mg

Cod And Mushrooms Mix

Servings: 4

Cooking Time: 25 Minutes

Ingredients:

- 2 cod fillets, boneless
- 4 tablespoons olive oil
- 4 ounces mushrooms, sliced
- Sea salt and black pepper to the taste
- 12 cherry tomatoes, halved
- 8 ounces lettuce leaves, torn
- 1 avocado, pitted, peeled and cubed
- 1 red chili pepper, chopped
- 1 tablespoon cilantro, chopped
- 2 tablespoons balsamic vinegar
- 1 ounce feta cheese, crumbled

Directions:

1. Put the fish in a roasting pan, brush it with 2 tablespoons oil, sprinkle salt and pepper all over and broil under medium-high heat for 15 minutes. Meanwhile, heat up a pan with the rest of the oil over medium heat, add the mushrooms, stir and sauté for 5 minutes.

2. Add the rest of the ingredients, toss, cook for 5 minutes more and divide between plates.

3. Top with the fish and serve right away.

Nutrition Info: calories 257, fat 10, fiber 3.1, carbs 24.3, protein 19.4

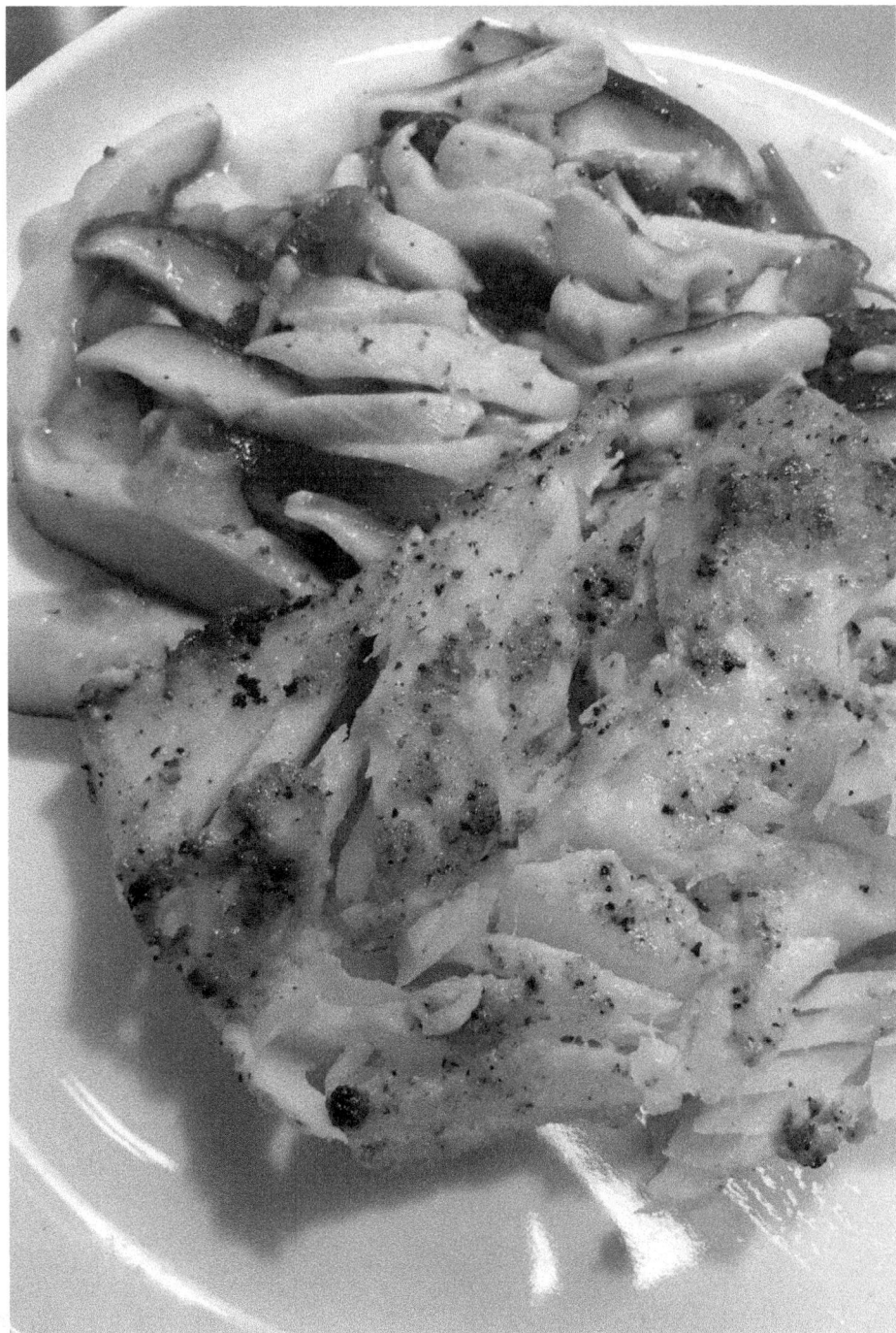

Baked Shrimp Mix

Servings: 4

Cooking Time: 32 Minutes

Ingredients:

- 4 gold potatoes, peeled and sliced
- 2 fennel bulbs, trimmed and cut into wedges
- 2 shallots, chopped
- 2 garlic cloves, minced
- 3 tablespoons olive oil
- ½ cup kalamata olives, pitted and halved
- 2 pounds shrimp, peeled and deveined
- 1 teaspoon lemon zest, grated
- 2 teaspoons oregano, dried
- 4 ounces feta cheese, crumbled
- 2 tablespoons parsley, chopped

Directions:

1. In a roasting pan, combine the potatoes with 2 tablespoons oil, garlic and the rest of the ingredients except the shrimp, toss, introduce in the oven and bake at 450 degrees F for 25 minutes.

2. Add the shrimp, toss, bake for 7 minutes more, divide between plates and serve.

Nutrition Info: calories 341, fat 19, fiber 9, carbs 34, protein 10

Lemon And Dates Barramundi

Servings: 2

Cooking Time: 12 Minutes

Ingredients:

- 2 barramundi fillets, boneless
- 1 shallot, sliced
- 4 lemon slices
- Juice of ½ lemon
- Zest of 1 lemon, grated
- 2 tablespoons olive oil
- 6 ounces baby spinach
- ¼ cup almonds, chopped
- 4 dates, pitted and chopped
- ¼ cup parsley, chopped
- Salt and black pepper to the taste

Directions:

1. Season the fish with salt and pepper and arrange on 2 parchment paper pieces.
2. Top the fish with the lemon slices, drizzle the lemon juice, and then top with the other ingredients except the oil.
3. Drizzle 1 tablespoon oil over each fish mix, wrap the parchment paper around the fish shaping to packets and arrange them on a baking sheet.

4. Bake at 400 degrees F for 12 minutes, cool the mix a bit, unfold, divide everything between plates and serve.

Nutrition Info: calories 232, fat 16.5, fiber 11.1, carbs 24.8, protein 6.5

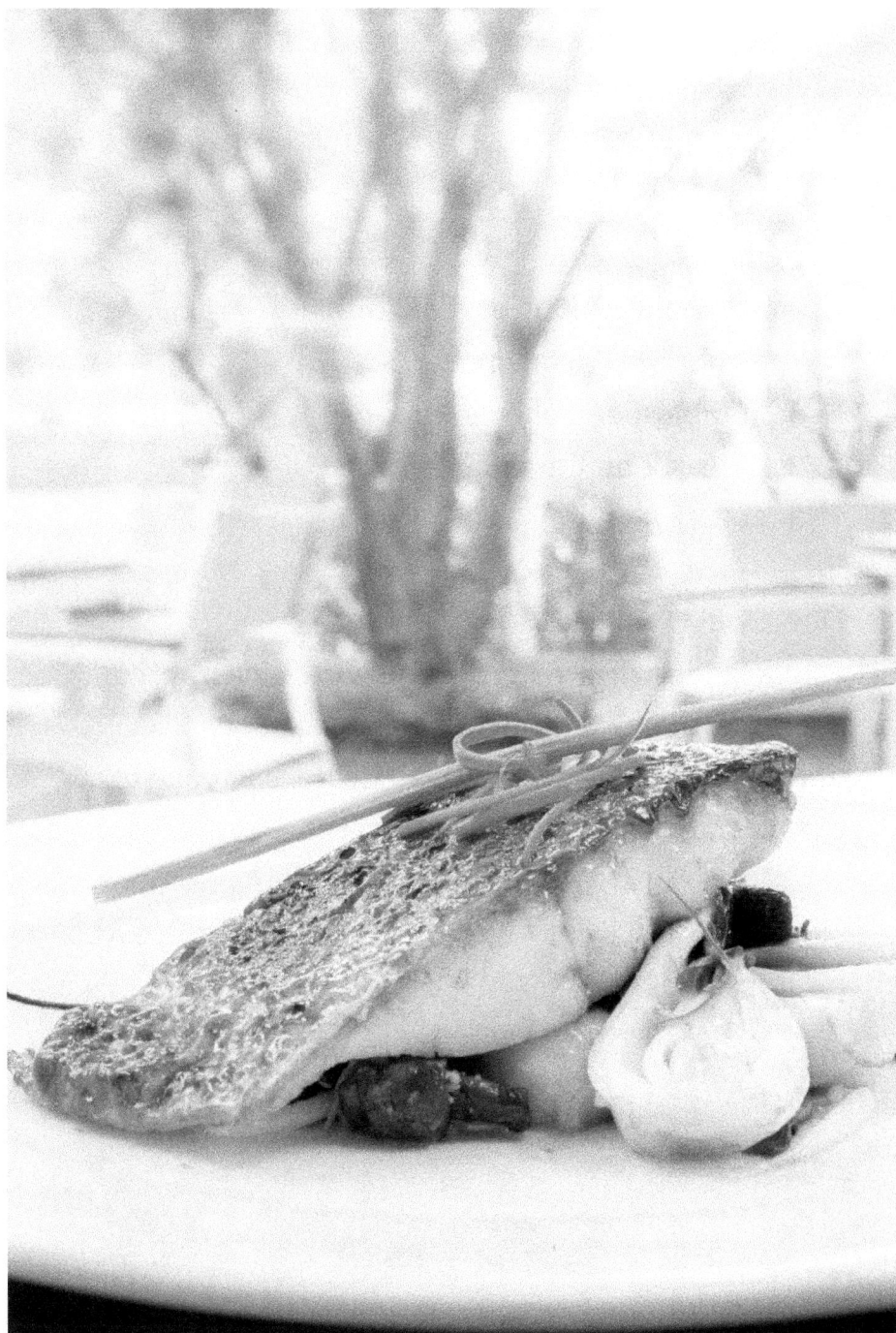

Cheesy Crab And Lime Spread

Servings: 8

Cooking Time: 25 Minutes

Ingredients:

- 1 pound crab meat, flaked
- 4 ounces cream cheese, soft
- 1 tablespoon chives, chopped
- 1 teaspoon lime juice
- 1 teaspoon lime zest, grated

Directions:

1. In a baking dish greased with cooking spray, combine the crab with the rest of the ingredients and toss.
2. Introduce in the oven at 350 degrees F, bake for 25 minutes, divide into bowls and serve.

Nutrition Info: calories 284, fat 14.6, fiber 5.8, carbs 16.5, protein 15.4

Honey Lobster

Servings: 2

Cooking Time: 10 Minutes

Ingredients:

- 2 lobster tails
- 2 teaspoons butter, melted
- 1 teaspoon honey
- ¼ teaspoon ground paprika
- 1 teaspoon lemon juice
- ¼ teaspoon dried dill

Directions:

1. Cut the top of the lobster tail shell to the tip of the tail with the help of the scissors. It will look like "lobster meat in a blanket".
2. Mix up together melted butter, honey, ground paprika, lemon juice, and dried dill.
3. Brush the lobster tails with butter mixture carefully from the top and down.
4. Preheat the oven to 365F.
5. Line the baking tray with parchment and arrange the lobster tails in it. 6. Bake the lobster tails for 10 minutes.

Nutrition Info:Per Serving:calories 91, fat 3.9, fiber 0.1 carbs 3.1, protein 0.1

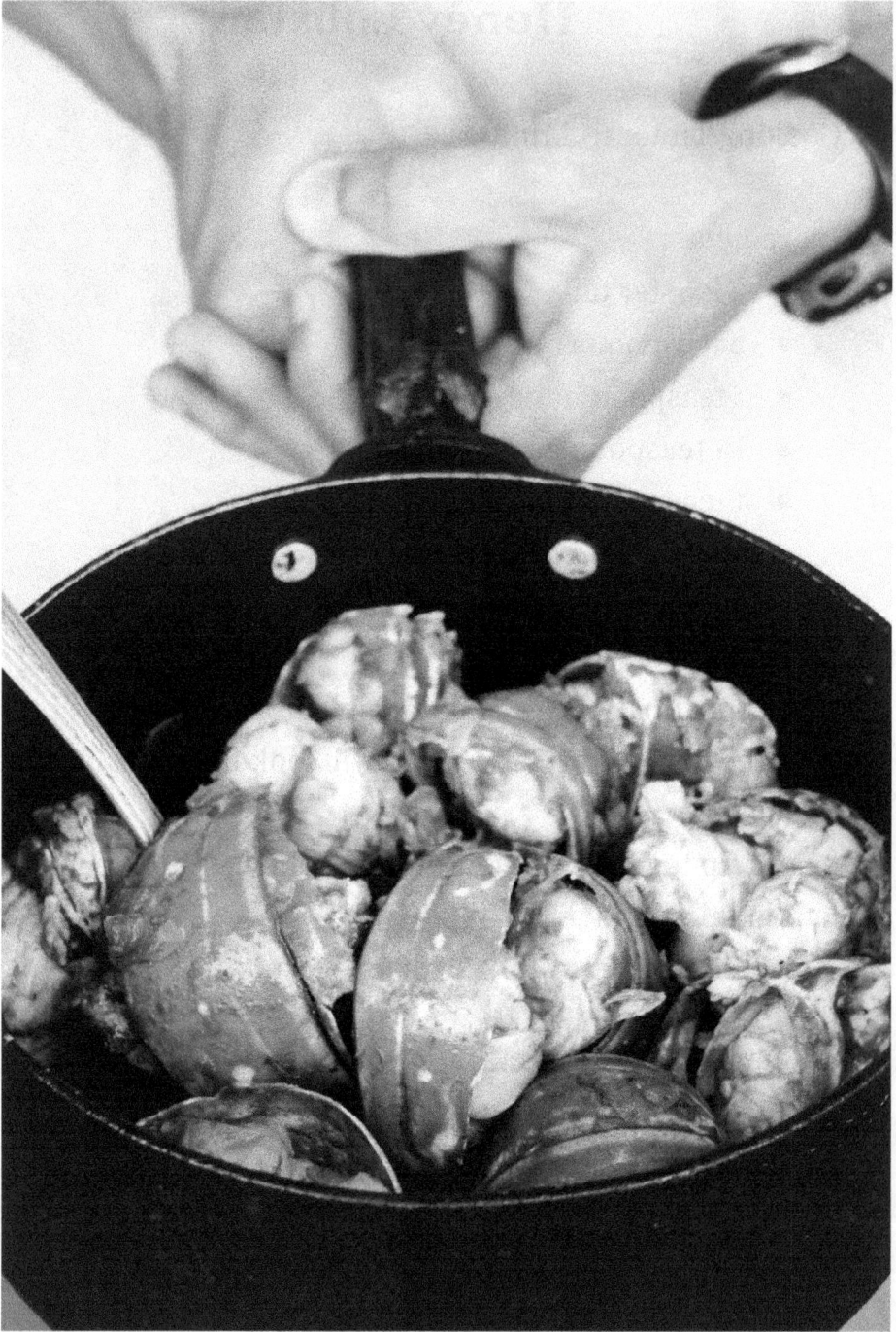

Fried Salmon

Servings: 2

Cooking Time: 8 Minutes

Ingredients:

- 5 oz salmon fillet
- ¼ teaspoon salt
- ½ teaspoon ground black pepper
- 1 tablespoon sunflower oil
- ¼ teaspoon lime juice

Directions:

1. Cut the salmon fillet on 2 lengthwise pieces.

2. Sprinkle every fish piece with salt, ground black pepper, and lime juice.

3. Pour sunflower oil in the skillet and preheat it until shimmering.

4. Then place fish fillets in the hot oil and cook them for 3 minutes from each side.

Nutrition Info:Per Serving:calories 157, fat 11.4, fiber 0.1, carbs 0.3, protein 13.8

Smoked Salmon And Veggies Mix

Servings: 4
Cooking Time: 20 Minutes

Ingredients:

- 3 red onions, cut into wedges
- ¾ cup green olives, pitted and halved
- 3 red bell peppers, roughly chopped
- ½ teaspoon smoked paprika
- Salt and black pepper to the taste
- 3 tablespoons olive oil
- 4 salmon fillets, skinless and boneless
- 2 tablespoons chives, chopped

Directions:

1. In a roasting pan, combine the salmon with the onions and the rest of the ingredients, introduce in the oven and bake at 390 degrees F for 20 minutes.
2. Divide the mix between plates and serve.

Nutrition Info: calories 301, fat 5.9, fiber 11.9, carbs 26.4, protein 22.4

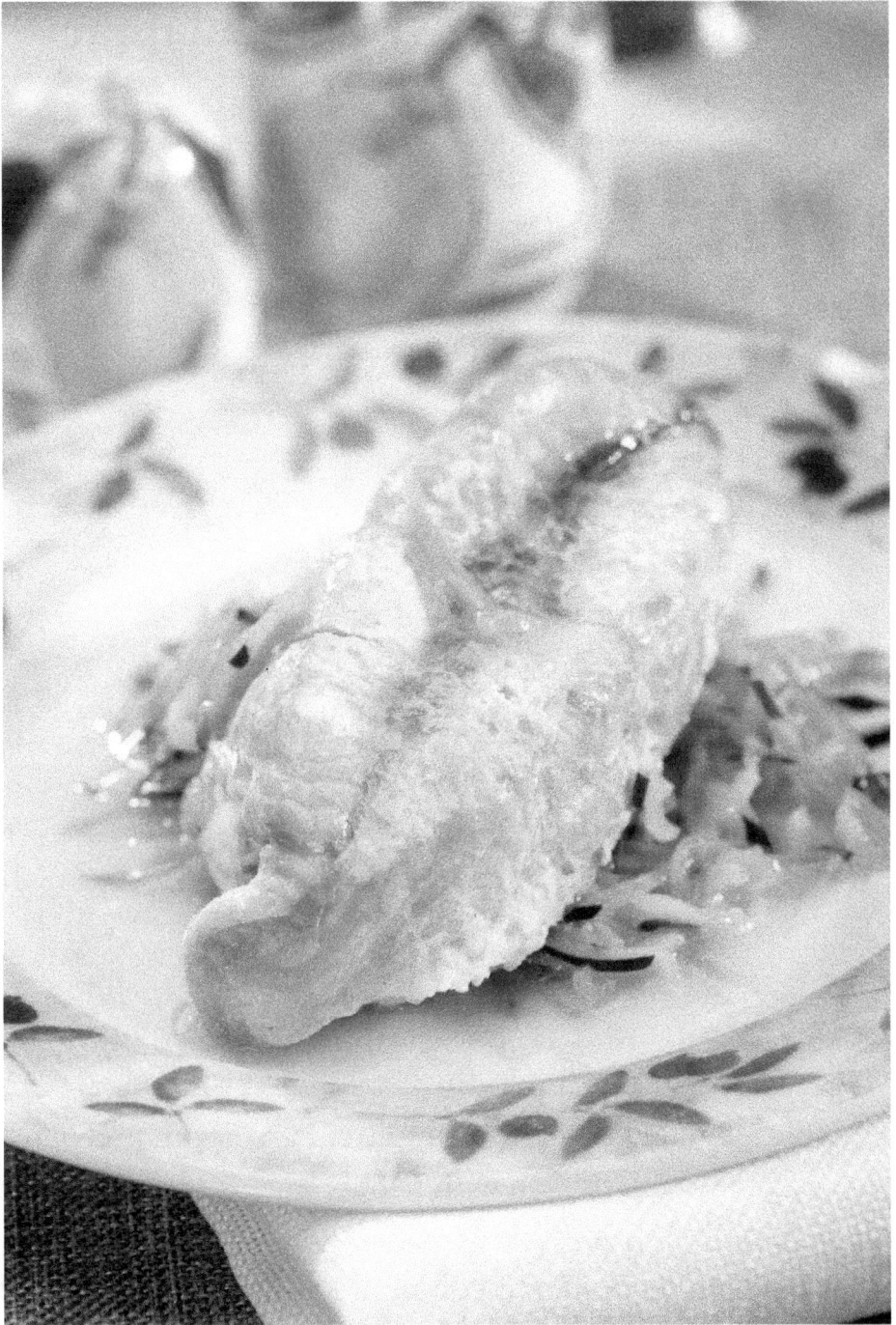

Berries And Grilled Calamari

Servings: 4

Cooking Time: 5 Minutes

Ingredients:

- ¼ cup dried cranberries
- ¼ cup extra virgin olive oil
- ¼ cup olive oil
- ¼ cup sliced almonds
- ½ lemon, juice
- ¾ cup blueberries
- 1 ½ pounds calamari tube, cleaned
- 1 granny smith apple, sliced thinly
- 1 tablespoon fresh lemon juice
- 2 tablespoons apple cider vinegar
- 6 cups fresh spinach
- Freshly grated pepper to taste
- Sea salt to taste

Directions:

1. In a small bowl, make the vinaigrette by mixing well the tablespoon of lemon juice, apple cider vinegar, and extra virgin olive oil. Season with pepper and salt to taste. Set aside.

2. Turn on the grill to medium fire and let the grates heat up for a minute or two.

3. In a large bowl, add olive oil and the calamari tube. Season calamari generously with pepper and salt.

4. Place seasoned and oiled calamari onto heated grate and grill until cooked or opaque. This is around two minutes per side.

5. As you wait for the calamari to cook, you can combine almonds, cranberries, blueberries, spinach, and the thinly sliced apple in a large salad bowl. Toss to mix.

6. Remove cooked calamari from grill and transfer on a chopping board. Cut into ¼-inch thick rings and throw into the salad bowl.

7. Drizzle with vinaigrette and toss well to coat salad.

8. Serve and enjoy!

Nutrition Info: Calories per Serving: 567; Fat: 24.5g; Protein: 54.8g; Carbs: 30.6g

Salmon And Zucchini Rolls

Servings: 8

Cooking Time: 0 Minutes

Ingredients:

- 8 slices smoked salmon, boneless
- 2 zucchinis, sliced lengthwise in 8 pieces
- 1 cup ricotta cheese, soft
- 2 teaspoons lemon zest, grated
- 1 tablespoon dill, chopped
- 1 small red onion, sliced
- Salt and pepper to the taste

Directions:

1. In a bowl, mix the ricotta cheese with the rest of the ingredients except the salmon and the zucchini and whisk well.

2. Arrange the zucchini slices on a working surface, and divide the salmon on top.

3. Spread the cheese mix all over, roll and secure with toothpicks and serve right away.

Nutrition Info: calories 297, fat 24.3, fiber 11.6, carbs 15.4, protein 11.6

Notes

www.ingramcontent.com/pod-product-compliance
Lightning Source LLC
Chambersburg PA
CBHW050757030426
42336CB00012B/1859